T0205859

Fundamentals of Evidence-Based Medicine

Kameshwar Prasad

Fundamentals of Evidence-Based Medicine

Second Edition

Springer

Kameshwar Prasad
Department of Neurology
Neurosciences Centre, and Clinical
Epidemiology Unit
All India Institute of Medical Sciences
New Delhi
Delhi
India

ISBN 978-81-322-1714-5 ISBN 978-81-322-0831-0 (eBook)
DOI 10.1007/978-81-322-0831-0
Springer India Heidelberg New York Dordrecht London

Printed on acid-free paper

Springer is part of Springer Science+Business Media (www.springer.com)

Dedicated to my dear parents, who left
for heavenly abode but continue to live
in our hearts and minds, and guide
us in all activities including writing this book

Foreword

In a perhaps apocryphal but certainly oft-quoted observation, a judge purportedly noted that while he couldn't define pornography, he knew it when he saw it. I feel in the same position when talking about genius.

I have observed, and admired, many excellent teachers of evidence-based medicine. There are very few, however, who I would say bring genius to their instruction. Kameshwar Prasad is one of those few. My first contact with Dr. Prasad was in 1992 while I was teaching one of the courses in our Clinical Epidemiology Master's program in which Dr. Prasad was enrolled. Since then, I've had the privilege, on many occasions, of watching Dr. Prasad teach. I've observed how he brings all the elements of any excellent instructor to his interaction with students. Engaging, enthusiastic, and deeply concerned about his learners, Dr. Prasad uses the techniques of small-group learning to motivate students to become fully involved in the process of discovery.

But that isn't genius. What differentiates Dr. Prasad from other outstanding teachers is his imagination in developing compelling examples that present complex concepts in simple ways. A potentially dry and difficult issue becomes an engaging story that draws the learners in and makes the educational process a pleasure. I have sat in classrooms listening to Dr. Prasad, and, as he started his story, I wondered, "Where is this guy going with this?" And in the end, there is revelation, and the climax of the story brilliantly illustrates some key point in understanding and interpreting the medical literature, and the science behind that literature.

As his teaching shares characteristics of other excellent teachers, Dr. Prasad's new text shares qualities with other top EBM texts. One sees excellent writing, logical flow, bite-sized messages, and clear and compelling format. EBM must be grounded in clinical practice, and Dr. Prasad makes superb use of clinical examples to illustrate EBM's fundamental principles. Visually oriented readers will find beautifully constructed tables that vividly summarize key issues. Those looking for further reading will not be overwhelmed with the references, but will find available suggestions for a small number of the best other resources. Those looking for sources of evidence to guide their practice will find the most practical of presentations: Resources are organized according to their cost. But what makes this book special is that Dr. Prasad's teaching genius, and the engaging, delightful personality behind that genius, comes through in the vivid, conversational writing style and, in particular, pedagogical techniques.

So, for instance, as you read this text, you will find a story of five friends getting together to decide who will get a free dinner that evening. You will be asked to consider how to interpret a prime ministerial popularity poll. You will learn how to evaluate the claims of two ultrasonographers, both of who claim to be able to tell you a baby's sex at 14 weeks gestation. You will find out how a Chair of an Accident and Emergency Department dealt with apparent overdiagnosis of appendicitis. These stories are often further enhanced by another brilliant technique: framing issues as conversations, and often conversations of discovery. So, reading this book, you will be exposed to dialogues between Dr. Prasad and his residents; between a neurologist and a neurosurgeon who disagree on the optimal management strategy; between a family doctor and a husband interested in his wife's expected date of delivery. In addition, we see amusing, imaginative and engaging mnemonic devices such as "Triple-E based medicine" or the three Cs of each of starting a study of therapy well, conducting it well, and finishing it well.

Additions in the second edition of this book both maintain Dr. Prasad's unique, engaging styles and add to both the more basic and more advanced parts of the text. The new chapter addressing 'formulating a focused clinical question' speaks to a fundamental EBM skill, while 'advanced topics' will delight the reader interested in cutting-edge EBM thinking. Dr. Prasad has also complemented the existing chapters with useful additions that carefully attend to the visual presentation of the material: Note, for instance, the 'forest plot' illustrating the meta-analysis chapter.

Reviews of books are not always just or insightful, and this is as true of medical texts as any other genre. In this case, however, justice has been done: The JAMA review of the first edition noted that students, residents as well as Master students of research methodology will find this book easy reading and very useful. While fitting, the JAMA comments represent an understatement: I don't think it is possible to have a clearer or more engaging presentation of the key concepts of EBM than the one Dr. Prasad offers. Readers of this book are in for a treat – and a learning experience that will leave them far better equipped to use the medical literature to improve their patient care.

Hamilton, ON, Canada Gordon Guyatt

Preface

The idea for this book came from repeated requests from the EBM workshop participants whom I had the privilege to work with. The workshops have taken place in India, Singapore, Oxford (UK), Bahrain, Oman, Saudi Arabia, Qatar, Egypt as well as Canada. The participants have somehow found my explanations more user-friendly and wanted to revisit these from time to time. It was because of this that I got motivated to write this book in a language that is simple to follow and easy to understand. I spent most of my leisure time during the last 3 years in writing this book.

My interest in evidence-based medicine started in 1992 when I, as an INCLEN (International Clinical Epidemiology Network) fellow, was pursuing the Master's degree in the Department of Clinical Epidemiology and Biostatistics at McMaster University, Hamilton, Canada. The degree was called 'Master in Design, Measurement and Evaluation of Health Care', but essentially it contained courses in critical appraisal, qualitative and quantitative research methods, meta-analysis, health economics, medical education and biostatistics. As a student, we were encouraged to attend the grand rounds of the department, and one of these rounds covered the topic of evidence-based medicine presented by Prof. Gordon Guyatt. Subsequently, in one of the Master courses, I had the privilege to be taught by Prof. Guyatt, who has served as my role model for all I do in the field of evidence-based medicine.

After my return to India in 1994, I had the privilege to share with Prof. Guyatt several teaching activities in EBM workshops which include the world-famous McMaster workshop on 'How to Teach Evidence-based Clinical Practice'. In all these activities, I have always learnt something new from Prof. Guyatt as well as the participants. During my stay in Bahrain for 3 years (2001–2004), I taught in more than 20 EBM workshops and directed the scientific activities of the International Gulf Reference Centre for evidence-based medicine at the College of Medicine and Medical Sciences, The Arabian Gulf University, Bahrain. I found each of the workshops useful in honing my teaching skills in EBM, and it is this experience that has shaped and reshaped many of the chapters of this book.

About This Book

A lot of material in this book is also available in other books [1, 2], and in fact, I have learnt a number of things that I write in this book from them. However, this book is different from all other books on evidence-based medicine in that there is greater emphasis on fundamental concepts. These concepts are presented in stories – some real, some imaginary. Each of the three main topics on therapy, diagnosis and meta-analysis start with a chapter on fundamental concepts and research process followed by a chapter on validity appraisal and then by a chapter on results appraisal. The chapter on prognosis combines all the three aspects in one. At the end, there are examples of critical appraisal of papers related to the various topics. Most of the critical appraisal questions are presented in three parts: Why do we ask the question? How do we find the answer? and How do we interpret the answer? I think this break-up helps in better understanding the process of critical appraisal. I must mention that you will find several repetitions of the same concept in different chapters but this is purposeful. I believe repetitions are helpful in understanding difficult concepts. I should also mention that this book avoids going deeper into the topics because the idea is to cover only the basic aspects. Those readers who want to delve deeper into the subject are referred to the manual by Prof. Guyatt and Dr. Rennie [3].

Who Should Read This Book?

I hope this book will be useful for all medical and nursing students, health-care professionals: doctors, nurses, dentists, physiotherapists and laboratory personnel. The laboratory personnel may find the chapters on diagnosis particularly useful. EBM has become one of the core knowledge and skills to be learnt in medical schools. Standards set by various agencies including World Federation of Medical Education require EBM skills to be taught in undergraduate as well as postgraduate medical education. The Accreditation Council of Graduate Medical Education in the USA has identified practice-based learning and improvement as one of the core competencies for residency training. This requires seeking literature for clinically relevant questions, appraising their validity and usefulness and applying it clinical practice.

The residents as well as medical and nursing students will find it helpful in searching health literature, assessing their value and applying the results in their practice. I hope the readers of this book enjoy it as much as I enjoyed writing it.

I warmly invite criticisms and comments that will improve the contents as well as format of this book. I welcome any suggestion to enhance the usefulness of this book to its readers.

New Delhi, India Kameshwar Prasad

References

1. Fletcher RH, Fletcher SW, Wagner EH, editors. Clinical epidemiology: the essentials. 3rd ed. Baltimore: Lippincott Wilkins & Company; 1996. p. 1–276.
2. Guyatt G, Rennie D, Meade M, Cook D, editors. Users' guides to the medical literature: a manual for evidence-based clinical practice, 2nd ed. (JAMA & Archives Journals). New York: McGraw-Hill Medical; 2008. p. 1–860.
3. Guyatt G, Rennie D, Meade M, Cook D, editors. Users' guides to the medical literature: essentials of evidence-based clinical practice, 2nd ed. (JAMA & Archives Journals). New York: McGraw-Hill Medical; 2008. p. 1–380.

Acknowledgement

I must begin by thanking the Rockefeller Foundation for training fellows like me in Clinical Epidemiology under the INCLEN programme. The fellowship afforded me the privilege to work with the wonderful faculty of the Department of Clinical Epidemiology and Biostatistics, McMaster University, Hamilton, Canada. There I received the training under the kind and erudite supervision of Prof. George Browman, the then chairman of the department. It was there in 1992 that I first heard the phrase 'evidence-based medicine' in one of the grand rounds presented by none other than Prof. Gordon Guyatt. Prof. Guyatt's elegant and persuasive presentation certainly initiated me into the field, and from then on, the journey continues. Several faculty members of the Department of Clinical Epidemiology and Biostatistics, McMaster University, Hamilton, Canada, have shaped my understanding and teaching of evidence-based medicine. However, I must specifically mention, besides Prof. Guyatt and Prof. Browman, Prof. Stephen Walter, Prof. Victor Neufeld, Prof. Brian Haynes, Prof. Roman Jaeschke, Prof. Chris Woodward and Prof. Salim Yusuf. Truly, the McMaster faculty formed the core of the international EBM working group led by Prof. Gordon Guyatt, who are the pioneers in the field.

I am greatly indebted to the All India Institute of Medical Sciences (AIIMS); Ministry of Health and Family Welfare, Government of India, New Delhi; College of Medicine and Medical Sciences (CMMS); the Arabian Gulf University (AGU), Bahrain; Ministry of Health, Bahrain; and the Bahrain Defence Force Hospital for providing me encouragement and opportunities to teach evidence-based medicine and hone my skills in teaching the subject. This book owes much to the stimulation and support of many of my colleagues at AIIMS as well as CMMS, AGU, particularly of Prof. Hossam Hamdy and Dr. Khaldoon Al-Roomi.

I acknowledge the contribution of the audiovisual unit of the Arabian Gulf University in helping prepare the diagrams in this book.

Last but not least, I have no words to express thanks to my wife, Meeta Prasad; my son, Kushagra Kumar; and my daughter, Manya Prasad, who have constantly encouraged and sometimes even cajoled me to finish writing this book as early as possible. I am grateful to them for sparing me in times of leisure and holidays that I spent writing this book rather than with them. Words particularly fail me in acknowledging the contribution of my wife Meeta Prasad who has watched over and taken care of me during all the activities related to EBM and writing of this book.

New Delhi, India Kameshwar Prasad

Contents

Chapter 1
Introduction to Evidence-Based Medicine

History

The term evidence-based medicine first appeared in 1990 in the information brochure for McMaster University Internal Medicine Residency Program. However, the work which led to its origin may be traced back to late 1970s, when Prof. David Sackett, the then Chairman of the Department of Clinical Epidemiology and Biostatistics McMaster University, Canada, published a series of articles in the *Canadian Medical Association Journal* beginning in 1981. The series was named 'The Readers' Guide to Medical Literature'. The series had one article devoted to each of the paper on diagnosis, treatment, prognosis, etc. The articles provided guides to critical appraisal of the various types of clinical papers. Internet did not exit at that time and information technology was in infancy. Not surprisingly, the series did not contain any section on 'how to search for relevant papers'.

The starting point was a journal paper at hand. The emphasis was on critical appraisal of the paper. The section on application. More than a decade had passed, when in early 1990s, a need was felt to re-visit and update the guides and include the latest advances in the field of critical appraisal. To do this, an international evidence-based medicine working group was formed at McMaster University, Canada. The group felt that the focus of the guides be changed from readers to users. The group thought that emphasis should be placed on usefulness of the information in clinical practice. The starting point may be a problem faced by the clinicians, who looks for relevant literature, finds it, critically appraises it and puts to use the information in his clinical practice. As sources of information had become enormous by then, and Internet had come into being, there was a need to guide the clinicians in searching the relevant literature. To incorporate these changes, the group worked to develop a series of papers (Users' Guides) to emphasise clinical practice and clinical decision-making based on sound evidence from clinical research [1]. During one of the retreats of the Department of Internal Medicine at McMaster University, one suggestion to name such clinical practice was to use the term 'scientific medicine', which was vehemently opposed by other members of the

K. Prasad, *Fundamentals of Evidence-Based Medicine*,
DOI 10.1007/978-81-322-0831-0_1, © Springer India 2013

department, mainly because of its implications that the practice so far had been 'unscientific'. Prof. Gordon Guyatt then suggested the term 'evidence-based medicine' which proved felicitous. He also chaired the working group and coedited the book 'User's Guide to Medical Literature'.

It would be unfair and plainly wrong to say that philosophical foundations of EBM originated in 1990s or even 1970s. In fact, it would be clear from the following discussions that the basic tenets had existed right from the inception of medical practice. All major civilisations may find some indications of some of its principles in their ancient texts and historical accounts.

What Is Evidence-Based Medicine?

In simple terms, it means using the current best evidence in decision-making in medicine in conjunction (together) with expertise of the decision-makers and expectations and values of the patients/people. The word medicine in EBM is often associated with doctors' profession, to distinguish EBM from evidence-based nursing or evidence-based public health, etc. Sometimes, people take even a narrower view and take medicine to mean internal medicine to distinguish EBM from evidence-based surgery, evidence-based dentistry, etc. But I take it in a broad sense to relate it to the health profession and distinguish it from other professions like law or business. In its broad sense, EBM becomes broader than evidence-based health care and includes public health, health policymaking, etc. While defining EBM, one should be clear what he means by medicine. Oxford dictionary defines medicine as a discipline for prevention and cure of disease. It is in this broad sense in which I use the term EBM.

EBM is a new paradigm of clinical practice and a process of lifelong learning, which emphasises a systematic and rigorous assessment of evidence for use in decision-making in health care in conjunction with expertise of the decision-makers and expectations and values of the patients.

Knowing About EBM (1-2-3-4)

Knowing EBM is like knowing 1-2-3-4. EBM has one goal, two fundamental principles, three components and four steps. *One goal* is to improve quality of clinical care; *two principles* are hierarchy of evidence and insufficiency of evidence alone in decision-making; *three components* are evidence, expertise and expectations of patients (triple Es); and *four steps* are ask, acquire, assess and apply (4 As). These are elaborated further in the following paragraphs.

Goal of EBM

EBM has one goal: to improve the health of people through decisions that will maximise their health-related quality of life and life span. The decisions may be in relation to public health, health care, clinical care, nursing care or health policy.

Principles of EBM

Two fundamental principles include:

(a) *Hierarchy of evidence*: It says that evidence available in any clinical decision-making can be arranged in order of strength based on likelihood of freedom from error. For example, for treatment decisions, meta-analyses of well-conducted large randomised trials may be the strongest evidence, followed in sequence by large multi-centric randomised trials, meta-analyses of well-conducted small randomised trials, single-centre randomised trials, observational studies, clinical experience or basic science research.
(b) *Insufficiency of evidence alone*: The second fundamental principle of EBM is that evidence alone is never sufficient for decision-making. It has to be integrated with clinical expertise and patients' expectations and values. This principle gives rise to considerations of components of EBM which follows below.

Components of EBM

In one sense, EBM is a misnomer, because besides evidence, two other Es are required for decision-making, namely:

(a) Expertise of the decision-makers
(b) Expectations and values of the patients/people

To emphasise all the three components, I use the word *Triple-E based medicine* (*TEBM*). To illustrate the importance of the two Es, other than evidence, two examples follow.

Example 1
A 28-year-old man is admitted to the intensive care unit with ascending paralysis and respiratory distress. The resident makes a diagnosis of Guillain–Barré syndrome (GBS) and starts to discuss evidence-based approaches to treat him. The consultant comes, takes history and suspects dumb rabies. It becomes clear that the patient had a dog bite 3 months ago and received only

partial immunisation. Further investigation confirmed the suspicion of dumb rabies, and the patient was shifted to Infectious Diseases Hospital for further treatment. The whole discussion on GBS was irrelevant. This example illustrates the role of expertise in practising EBM. If the diagnosis is wrong, all the EBM discussion is superfluous.

Example 2
Expectations, values and circumstances of the patients/people:

(a) The diagnosis of motor neurone disease (amyotrophic lateral sclerosis) requires certain level of expertise and experience. Once the diagnosis is made, one can look for evidence in favour of certain treatments like riluzole. It turns out that there is definitive evidence from RCTs and meta-analysis indicating that riluzole can prolong tracheostomy – free life for 3 months if taken regularly (usually for years). The cost of riluzole treatment is prohibitive. In view of the high cost and risk of hepatotoxicity (and the need to pay out of pocket in India), many neurologists and their patients do not use this. Patients do not consider it 'worth it'; however, some patients who can easily afford to take riluzole for the treatment of this condition are prescribed with this drug.

(b) There is a consistent evidence to show that alcohol in moderation is protective against heart attacks and stroke. However, in Islam, alcohol is forbidden. It would be unacceptable to discuss alcohol intake in moderation with a staunch Muslim even if he has many risk factors for heart attack and stroke.

Goal of EBM	Improve health of people through high-quality health care
Principles of EBM	Evidence has a hierarchy
	Evidence alone is not enough
Components of EBM (3 Es)	Evidence
	Expertise
	Expectations
Steps of EBM (4 As)	Ask, acquire, assess, apply

Why EBM?

The above examples indicate the need to integrate expertise and patients' values with the evidence in clinical decision-making. This is what practice of evidence-based medicine requires. You might ask – isn't it what physicians always did and ought to do? How else did we make health-care decisions? Well, there have been a number of different bases for such decisions other than evidence. The examples below are mainly for clinical decisions, but similar examples for policy decisions can also be cited.

Physiologic Rationale

On many occasions, we make a decision on the basis of physiologic or pathophysiologic rationale. For example, ischaemic stroke is commonly due to occlusion of middle cerebral artery (MCA). It makes physiologic sense to bypass the occlusion by connecting some branch of the external carotid to a branch of MCA beyond the occlusion. Such on operation is called external carotid–internal carotid (EC–IC) bypass. Based on this rationale, thousands of EC–IC bypass surgeries were being performed in many parts of the world, until some people questioned it. An international trial sponsored by NIH (USA) compared this to medical treatment and showed that the surgery is not only ineffective but also delays recovery [2]. After this evidence was published, the number of EC–IC bypass surgeries crashed in North America and is rarely, if ever, performed for ischaemic stroke anywhere in the world.

A second example is use of streptokinase, a thrombolytic agent, in ischaemic stroke. It makes physiologic sense to use streptokinase to dissolve the clot in this condition (just as in myocardial infarction). But three clinical trials (known as MAST-E,[1] MAST- I[2] and ASK[3]) had to be stopped prematurely because more patients were dying with the use of streptokinase than without it. As a result, streptokinase is not used for ischaemic stroke, but surprisingly, tissue plasminogen activator (t-PA), another thrombolytic agent, is associated with less increase in mortality and overall better outcome, though physiologically, we do not know any good reason for this difference.

Several other examples (like increased mortality with encainide as antiarrhythmic agent) show that physiologically reasonable decisions may have unacceptable clinical risk and, therefore, clinical studies are necessary to determine the benefit–risk profile. Decisions based solely on physiologic rationale may cause more harm than good.

Experts' Advice

We often seek experts' advice to take certain treatment decisions. Policymakers often seek experts' advice to take a policy decision. However, experts' advice without reference to adequate search and evaluation of evidence may be simply wrong.

Take example of treatment of eclampsia. A survey conducted in UK in 1992 showed that only 2 % of obstetricians used magnesium sulphate to control

---

[1] Multicentre Acute Stroke Trial – Europe
[2] Multicentre Acute Stroke Trial – Italy
[3] Australian Streptokinase Trial

convulsions in eclampsia. The preferred drug was diazepam. I have personally seen neurologists advising use of diazepam rather than magnesium sulphate. But evidence from clinical trials showed clearly that magnesium sulphate is more effective in not only controlling convulsions but also decreasing maternal mortality in eclampsia [3]. It is reassuring to note that in England the Royal College of Obstetrics and Gynaecology recently adopted the recommendation to use magnesium sulphate, rather than diazepam in this condition.

Textbooks and Reviewers

We often look into textbooks or review articles for deciding to use an intervention. A number of examples are available to show that textbooks or review articles may recommend to use potentially harmful intervention and may not recommend to use potentially (or even established) helpful intervention. A classic example of this is streptokinase (SK) in acute myocardial infarction (AMI). Lau et al [4] have shown that had there been a periodically updated summary of emerging evidence (called 'cumulative meta-analysis'), a strong case for recommending routine use of SK in AMI could be made in 1977 but even in 1982, 12 out of 13 articles did not mention SK for AMI (one mentioned it as an experimental drug). Recommendation became common (15 out of 24 articles) only near 1990, almost 13 years after there was enough clinical evidence.

On the other hand, most textbook/review articles in 1970 were recommending routine use of lignocaine hydrochloride in acute MI (in nine out of 11 articles), whereas evidence to date was showing a trend towards increased mortality with its use. It was only after 1989 when evidence summary in the form of meta-analysis was published that textbooks and review articles stopped recommending its use in AMI.

Manufacturers' Claims

Many clinicians often start using an intervention based on the information from the drug companies. However, the information may not be valid and may result in more harm than good. An example is the use of hormone replacement therapy (HRT) in postmenopausal women. The companies promoted the use of HRT without adequate and high-quality evidence. Only when a large clinical trial showed that it may be dangerous that the clinicians have stopped recommending HRT widely [5].

Many clinicians are easily convinced by drug company information, though many a times it may be misleading.

The above examples show that decisions based exclusively on pathophysiologic rationale, experts' advice, textbook/review articles or drug company information may turn out to be wrong. This is not to say that all the time they are wrong or that

Table 1.1 Concepts or notions before and after introduction of EBM

	Pre-EBM notions/concepts	EBM notions/concepts
1. Clinical/medical education	Is sufficient to practice EBM	Necessary but not sufficient Need lifelong, self-directed learning and reflective practice
2. Clinical experience	Sufficient to guide practice	Necessary but not sufficient Needs to be aware of research results
3. Textbooks and review (traditional) articles	Are sufficient	Useful but not sufficient Often need to refer to systematic review/original research
4. Medline	Is the resource of first resort	Medline is a resource of last resort
5. Evidence from basic and animal research	Is adequate to guide clinical practice	Necessary but not sufficient Needs clinical evidence
6. Validity of publications	All that is published (in top journals) is largely true (unless contradicted by another publication)	Most of what is published (even in top journals) is largely untrue
7. Reading conclusions of paper	Is sufficient	Necessary but not sufficient Need to read methods and results
8. Critical appraisal ability	Comes automatically and informally with medical education and experience	Needs to be learnt actively and formally
9. Statistical significance	Statistical significance is sufficient	Necessary but not sufficient Needs to assess clinical significance

advice based on a clinical trial or meta-analysis cannot go wrong. But the point is that when physiologic rationale or experts' advice is supported by clinical evidence, the likelihood of such decisions going wrong is lower than when they are not supported by the evidence. When there is discrepancy between the above sources, then there is a need to exercise caution and put more weight on valid clinical evidence than on other bases. EBM puts emphasis on this point.

What Is New in EBM?

It may be argued that physicians (or health policymakers) have always used and continue to use evidence, expertise and patients' values in decision-making. Yes, this is largely true. All good physicians always did it and continue to do it. The new thing is the difference in emphasis, explicitness, rigour and understanding. The new tools and techniques of accessing, appraising and expressing the evidence make the process (of using evidence) more systematic and rigorous. Many notions and concepts carried by physicians before EBM era need to be changed. Some of such notices or concepts are given in Table 1.1.

Steps in Practising EBM

The main (but not the only) objective of EBM is the application of the right and complete *information* by health-care professionals in decision-making. To meet this objective, four key steps (4 As) are necessary:

(a) Ask for the required information by formulating your question.
(b) Acquire (find) the information by searching resources.
(c) Assess or appraise the relevance, quality and importance of the information.
(d) Apply the information in your practice or patient.

Each of the above steps is outlined below:

Step 1: Asking for the Required Information in the Form of a Question

Asking question in a particular format is an important first step, because it helps to find the most relevant information. It specifies the outcomes you are looking for. It also helps in assessing the relevance of the information to your patient's problem.

Literally, hundreds of questions may be asked in relation to a patient's problem. The questions may pertain to anatomy, physiology, pathology, epidemiology, diagnosis, treatment or pharmacology – to name a few. The questions can be classified into two types:

(a) *General (background) questions*: those related to anatomy, physiology, biochemistry, pathology, pharmacology, diagnostic approach, general management, etc.
(b) *Focused (foreground) questions*: those related to interpretation of a specific diagnostic test, risk and benefits of a particular treatment and a given patient's prognosis.

The Table 1.2 gives the differences between the two sets of questions.

Table 1.2 Differences between general (background) and specific (foreground) questions

	General (background)	Focused (foreground)
Activities to relate to	Knowing basic sciences like anatomy and pathophysiology	Patient care, often of an individual patient
Who asks?	Mostly students	Mostly experienced physicians
Example 1: Diagnosis of early pregnancy	What are the clinical features and tests available for diagnosis of early pregnancy?	What is the sensitivity and specificity of ultrasound in the diagnosis of early pregnancy?
Example 2: Treatment of Guillain–Barré syndrome (GBS)	What are the available options for treatment for GBS?	What are the risks and benefits of steroids in the treatment of GBS, particularly in this patient?
Example 3: Prognosis of GBS	What are the prognostic factors in GBS?	What is the prognosis of this patient with GBS?

Sources of the Questions

The questions arise in our day-to-day practice on almost daily basis. In fact, many questions may arise every day. You may be on rounds – seeing a patient with post-traumatic vertigo. One of your colleagues asks – why not start him on a vasodilator? You may be seeing patients in outpatient department. Your patient with migraine may ask – is there any herbal remedy for my problem? What about acupuncture? You may be in a seminar. Your colleague challenges the superiority of laparoscopic appendectomy over mini-laparotomy. You may yourself wonder at times whether there is any point in doing MRI in this patient with stroke, whether 3-D ultrasound will alter my management of this patient with pregnancy and so on.

You will face such questions every day that require and motivate you to seek evidence from literature. However, it is important not to rush to the Internet without some deeper thinking. I have seen some residents coming up with a paper, which bears superficial resemblance to the question but has nothing to do with it. Deeper thinking leads to refinement of the question.

Refining the Question

We discussed a patient with stroke in our round. One of my residents asked: Why are we not giving heparin to this patient? I said, it would be better if you yourself find the answer to the question and share with the whole department in the next journal club. She agreed.

The following conversation between my resident and myself illustrates the importance of refining the question:

I: Where will you look for the evidence?
R: My first choice would be Cochrane Library. Isn't it right?
I: Yes, that is right. But what is your question precisely?
R: Well, what is the role of heparin in acute stroke?
I: Which type of stroke are you talking about?
R: Clearly, ischaemic stroke?
I: Ischaemic stroke occurs in young patients with rheumatic heart disease. Are you interested in papers with such patients?
R: No, no. In elderly patients. My patient is 65 years old.
I: Even in elderly patients some have non-valvular atrial fibrillation or other cardiac disease and stroke. Would you look for papers with such patients?
R: But my patient does not have any such disease. I would like to focus on atherothrombotic cerebral infarctions.
I: So, can you restate your question?
R: What is the role of heparin in elderly patients with atherothrombotic ischaemic stroke (infarctions)?
I: That's better. But tell me are you interested in standard heparin or low molecular weight heparin?
R: Any heparin

I: O.K., but what are you looking for - Recovery or prevention of recurrence of stroke? You will find reviews looking at recovery from acute attack or at prevention of recurrence of stroke or both. Which outcome are you interested in?
R: I am interested in recovery from acute attack.
I: How do you define recovery?
R: Well, recovery means recovery. Patient regains his pre-stroke functional status.
I: What about recovery to a point that he is able to do his activities of daily living independently. Will you consider it an important recovery?
R: Yes, that is acceptable.
I: Can you restate your question now?
R: In elderly patients with acute ischaemic stroke, does heparin improve the chances of recovery, defined as independence in activities of daily living?
I: That's better. One final wrinkle. Are you comparing heparin with no-heparin or heparin vs. aspirin?
R: I am not sure. Our patient is already on aspirin. Therefore, my question would be what if we add heparin to aspirin, which means aspirin plus heparin vs. aspirin alone. But I would also look at studies which compare heparin to aspirin or heparin without aspirin vs. no heparin, no aspirin.
I: That means you have three questions.
R: Yes, my type of patient and outcomes are one set but there are three sets of interventions.
I: Isn't it something like this?

Patients	Elderly with acute ischaemic stroke due to atherothrombosis		
Interventions	Aspirin plus heparin	Heparin, no aspirin	Heparin, no aspirin
Comparison	Aspirin alone	Aspirin	No heparin, no aspirin
Outcome	Full recovery or independence in activities of daily living		

R: Yes, that's what I want.

This dialogue illustrates the need to think deeper and formulate your question with some level of specificity; otherwise, you may pick up an irrelevant paper, and you may waste a lot of time in shuffling through a lot of irrelevant papers. However, I must say that you should not be too specific; otherwise, you risk finding no paper. You may start with moderate specificity and depending on the number of 'hits' found in your search, you may increase or decrease the level of specificity and adjust your search to get a manageable number of papers.

To summarise, you need to specify the following in your clinical questions:

(a) Patient population: type of patients
(b) Intervention (new): the new approach or strategy of treatment
(c) Comparison: the control intervention
(d) Outcomes: clinically meaningful outcomes that are important for the patients

The acronym 'PICO' is used to memorise the parts of a well-formulated clinical question. I must say that sometimes the comparison intervention may be missing, and 'PIO' is enough to specify the question.

Beginners face difficulty in deciding which intervention goes under 'I' and which one under 'C'. 'I' stands for the new intervention. To emphasise this, I use the acronym 'PInCO' where 'n' by the side of I stands for new.

The above discussion illustrates that formulating a good clinical question is not simple. Certain level of experience is necessary to optimally specify the patients, interventions and outcomes. Only the experienced professionals can specify the outcomes, which are clinically meaningful in a particular context.

Step 2: Acquiring (Searching for) the Evidence (see Chap. 2)

Step 3: Assessment or Critical Appraisal of the Papers

There are four issues in the critical appraisal:

(a) Relevance
(b) Validity
(c) Consistency
(d) Importance or significance of results

(a) Relevance refers to the extent to which the research paper matches your information need. Comparing the research question in the paper with your clinical question would help you to determine the relevance of the paper. Once again, PICO format of the question would make it easy to take the decision. Many a times, you may find a match between the population and/or intervention, but the outcomes are different. Unless you find another paper with the desired outcomes, it may be advisable to proceed with the paper.
(b) Validity refers to the extent to which the results are free from bias. Biases are mainly of three types:

    1. Selection bias
    2. Measurement bias
    3. Bias in analysis (In all types of studies, you must look for these biases. The specific questions are given in Table 1.3.)

All kinds of studies need to be assessed for the above biases, while assessing validity. If a bias is present, you should ask the next question – so what? Does it affect the internal validity or external validity? Let me briefly explain what these terms mean?

1. Internal validity is concerned with the question: Are the results correct for the subjects in the study? This is the primary or first question for any study.
2. External validity asks the question: To which population are the results of the study applicable or generalisable? External validity is judged in terms of time, place and person. Can the results be extrapolated to the current or future time, to different geographical region or settings and to patients outside the study?

Table 1.3 PICO format of clinical questions

	Therapy	Diagnosis	Prognosis	Meta-analysis (systematic research of a study of studies)
Selection bias	Are the patients selected into the groups prognostically similar?	Do the patients represent wide spectrum of the disease	Do the patients represent wide spectrum of the disease?	Were studies selected exhaustively and reproducibly?
Measurement bias A. Missing (incomplete measurement)	Was follow-up complete?	Did everyone get both the new test and the gold standard (no verification bias)	Was follow-up complete?	Is there publication bias?
B. Outcome measurement	Was outcome assessment done by blinded observers?	Were the doers of the new test and the gold standard blinded to each other's results?	Was the outcome assessment objective and unbiased (without being aware of the presence or absence of the prognostic factors)	Was data abstraction done by (at least) two observers independently? What is the level of agreement between the two?
Bias in analysis	Was analysis based on intention-to-treat principle?			Were results similar from study to study?

Internal validity is the basic requirement of a study. However, it is an ideal to aspire for. It is nearly impossible to achieve 100 % internal validity and many attempts to maximise internal validity may compromise the external validity. A reasonable balance needs to be achieved between internal and external validity.

(c) Consistency refers to the extent to which the research results are similar across different analyses in the study and are in agreement with evidence outside the study. Consistency may be internal or external.

1. *Internal consistency* looks at the different analyses conducted in the study. For example, in a therapy paper there may be unadjusted and adjusted analysis, certain sensitivity analyses, analyses for subgroups and analyses of primary and secondary outcomes. If these analyses yield the same answer, say, in favour of the new treatment, then the results will be considered internally consistent.
2. *External consistency* refers to the consistency of study's findings with the evidence from biology, from other studies and even with the experience of clinicians. If findings are not consistent with one or more of these, one needs to explore the reasons. Knowledge of biology is vast, evolving and yet (to a great extent) incomplete. Hence, most of the time some biological explanations can always be found to explain the results. If not, one should remember the limit of our knowledge of human biology.

(d) Significance of the information (results): This needs to be evaluated in the light of the type of paper. For therapy (treatment) and diagnosis (test) paper, you need to ask:

1. How did the new treatment or test perform in the study? Were the results statistically significant and clinically important?
2. What information can you take from the study to your practice/patient?

Step 4: Applying the Results to Your Patient

Having found that the information in the paper is relevant, valid, consistent and important, the question is whether the test or treatment will be useful for your patient/practice. You need to determine (or best guess) your patient's disease probability or risk of adverse outcome and then consider how these will change with the application of the new test or treatment. Whether this change is worth the risk and cost of the new interventions?

What does your patient think about the benefits and risks associated with the new test or treatment? These considerations would help you to apply (or not to apply) the results of the paper and take a decision. A practice which is based on these considerations is aptly called 'evidence-based clinical practice'.

EBM as a Strategy

EBM is a strategy to solve problems, to learn effectively and efficiently, to empower learners and decision-makers, to avoid wasteful expenditures and to improve quality of health care.

Towards Quality of Care Improvement

1. *A problem-solving strategy*: a clinical practitioner or a policymaker faces problems almost every day. The clinician has to make a decision to prescribe a diagnostic test or a treatment. The policymaker has to decide whether to purchase a technology. They need information to make the decision. Often this information helps to judge the utility of the treatment or technology. They need to search this information and assess its validity, meaning and applicability in their context. EBM provides the skills to efficiently search and assess the information so that it can be used to solve the problems.
2. *An empowering strategy*: EBM empowers patients by clarifying whether there is evidence clearly in favour of one intervention or another or that evidence is unclear and, therefore, the patient's preferences would count more in the decision-making. EBM empowers junior doctors and nurses or even students by providing opportunities for them to support their contention with evidence rather than blindly following their seniors.
3. *A waste limiting strategy*: By raising questions about the evidence of benefits and risks or costs about several routine procedures, EBM has the potential to reduce wasteful expenditures. For example, routine liver function tests in all cases of stroke is challenged by lack of evidence of any benefit and may be dropped leading to savings for the patients as well as hospitals.
4. *A quality improvement strategy*: Quality requires maximisation of benefits and risks for the patients. It requires organisational and individual learning. It requires guidelines and review criteria based on evidence. It encourages limiting wasteful expenditures. It is based on the philosophy of empowerment of workers. As indicated above, EBM helps in all of these and hence is a strategy to improve quality of health care.
5. *A protective strategy against misleading information*: Sometimes, probably very often, manufacturers of drugs and devices provide potentially misleading information to health professionals and make taller claim than justified. EBM makes the professionals wary of such claims and protects them from prescribing drugs and procedures with unsubstantiated claims. It gives them skills to judge the appropriateness of such claims.
6. *A communication facilitating strategy*: Health professionals often differ in their approach and opinion while dealing with a patient problem. In the ever-growing need for a teamwork and multidisciplinary approach to patient care, communication is a key to success. The opinions may differ because of differences in the evidence base or values that go into decision-making. EBM provides skills to delineate the basis of differing opinion and a language to communicate with colleagues, with explicit description of evidence and values.

7. *A learning strategy*: Medical educators espouse self-directed lifelong learning for health professionals. But how to achieve this? EBM offers at least one way of achieving this. By being relevant to one's practice, EBM is consistent with the principles of adult learning.

Towards Education

8. *An information handling strategy*: It is estimated that more than two million articles are published annually in more than 20,000 journals. It is impossible for anyone to read all of them. Health professionals may be overwhelmed and bewildered if asked to read all of them. It is important to separate the insignificant and unsound studies from salient and crucial or to know the right sources that would have done this. Efficiency and selectivity are of crucial importance. EBM provides the basis for this efficiency and selectivity.
9. *A collaborative learning strategy*: There is increasing emphasis in medical education nowadays for collaborative and inter-professional learning. EBM is a common ground and base on which all health professionals may collaborate in learning.

Towards Research

10. A research promotion strategy: EBM process includes accessing and appraising research. The process often leads to identification of shortcomings in existing research and awareness of lack of good research in a topic or field. This may become a starting point for many residents and practitioners to plan and conduct research. The process also leads to awareness of many terms and concepts which help in understanding research methodology and motivate people to take further steps to plan a good research in the area where no sound evidence exists.

Limitations of EBM

1. *Limited applicability of evidence to an individual patient*: The evidence that is most applicable to a patient is the one coming from a study on him alone. Such studies are possible and are usually termed, N-of-1 trials. If the patient can be treated with a drug and a placebo in random order and effects can be measured, the results will be very applicable to him. But the scope of such studies is very limited. Only chronic conditions with repeatable outcomes (unlike MI, stroke or death) are suitable for such studies. Moreover, most health-care professionals do not have time, facility or inclination to conduct studies. Therefore, the evidence, which is available, comes from averaging over a number of patients, some of whom had beneficial effects, some had adverse effects and some had both. Is this average effect applicable to your patient? You don't know, you can't know. This is probably the biggest limitation of EBM. But what is the alternative? To have some idea of what happens on average is usually better than having no idea at all.

The average effect is what would happen to most of your patients. In the absence of a better alternative, this is probably the best knowledge to work with.

2. *Lack of consistent and coherent evidence*: This is another big problem. For many questions that are encountered in clinical practice, there is little evidence, certainly very little good evidence. For many questions, evidence is available but inconsistent and incoherent. Recent controversy on effectiveness of mammography for breast cancer exemplifies the incoherence, which afflicts some of the available evidence.
3. *Potential to limit creativity and innovation*: EBM puts the standards of proof at such a high level that a new idea may be crushed even before sprouting. For example, if a new test is developed to diagnose, say migraine or tension headache, the investigators may feel limited in conducting a good study because there is no 'gold standard', which is highlighted (even though, not true) as a 'must' by the current EBM literature.
4. *Need for time from clinicians*: Clinicians are busy everywhere, more so in developing countries. The time required to learn even the language of EBM is not available. This poses a major limitation for the clinicians, even to read and understand pre-appraised EBM literature.
5. *Limited availability of EBM resources*: Many of the EBM resources, particularly secondary ones, are not available or affordable by clinicians, particularly in developing countries. Even local libraries do not carry them. Many clinicians may not have computers or Internet access. Under the circumstances, the clinicians cannot access the literature and thus cannot practice EBM. Also the human resource and expertise necessary for promoting EBM are limited at present.
6. *Need to learn new concepts* (methodological and statistical): Many concepts in EBM are difficult to learn. One or two workshops are not enough to clarify those concepts. This puts many clinicians off. They develop a kind of aversion towards EBM.
7. *Confusing terminology*: Many new terms which have been created by EBM proponents are unnecessary and confusing. Simple and self-explanatory terms like risk difference and risk ratio have been called absolute risk reduction and relative risk, respectively. Similarly, incidence of an outcome in control group has been termed in EBM books as risk in control group and also as control event rate (which strictly speaking is not a rate). These duplicate terms confuse clinicians who, as such, are not comfortable with numbers and mathematics.
8. *Wrong assumptions*: EBM books and articles nearly always assume that risk ratios of treatments and likelihood ratios of diagnostic test results are more or less constant across patient subgroups and apply even to individuals. In fact, these assumptions have often been found to be wrong. Of course these measures are more stable across patient subgroups than other measures, but that they are stable across subgroups of patients or across different population of patients is untrue. Yet, these are fundamental assumptions on which EBM rests.

Misconceptions About EBM

1. *Patient waits while the doctor searches and appraises the evidence*: Sometimes, critics cite instances from emergency that cannot wait while the doctor is looking for evidence. But this is a misconception. Urgent decisions have to be taken based on what the doctor knows or gathers from other colleagues who are involved in the care of the patient. However, if he has a question, evidence to which he is uncertain about, he follows the four steps of EBM whenever time permits. He may change his decision after knowing the evidence. It is expected that physicians would be up to date about the evidence involving commonly encountered conditions, particularly the emergencies, and won't have to start an EBM process while the patient waits for action in the emergency.
2. *Clinical expertise is ignored in EBM*: Nothing can be farther than the truth than what this statement suggests. On the contrary, expertise and experience are essential to practice EBM. Without these, even the first step of asking the question cannot begin. Specifying the clinically meaningful outcomes requires some clinical expertise. Similarly, evaluation of a 'gold standard' in diagnosis and baseline prognostic balance, post-randomisation withdrawals from analysis. In therapy requires expert judgment. Thus, rather than ignoring, EBM emphasises integrating one's clinical expertise and experience with evidence.
3. *Only randomised trials or meta-analyses are counted as 'evidence'* – Most criticisms against EBM have been mainly criticisms of randomised trials and meta-analyses, as if only the latter are counted as evidence. This is not true. Read any book on EBM, you will find that it counts clinical experience, observational studies, basic research as well as animal studies as evidence. What EBM asserts is that strength of evidence varies as regards its validity, clinical applicability and adequacy for benefit – risk analysis. Randomised evidence is often stronger for these purposes than other kinds of evidence. At times, though, clinical experience may be the dominant factor in decision-making.For example consider a patient with subarachnoid haemorrhage and wide-neck berry aneurysm. Suppose evidence suggests that coiling is the best option, but the clinical team has no experience of this. The neurosurgeon may reasonably decide to do carotid ligation in view of urgency and his experience.There are many disorders for which nonrandomised evidence is the most acceptable level of evidence and nobody has ever asked for randomised trials. For example, for all deficiency disorders (e.g. hypokalemia, hypothyroidism), replacement therapy is well accepted based on observational studies alone. To my knowledge, nobody has ever asked a randomised trial for these and for many other endocrine and haematological disorders, though questions like tight versus loose control of diabetes did need randomised evidence.
4. *EBM is a method for medical research*: Many participants in EBM workshops come with an idea that they are going to learn clinical research methods. This is a misconception. EBM is for users of research. Doing research requires a greater

involvement and deeper knowledge. EBM workshops last from few days to 1 week. The time may be adequate only for understanding the language of EBM, not even for inculcating ability to do independent critical appraisal of literature. EBM intends to make practitioners more informed users of research.

References

1. Guyatt GH, Rennie D. Users' guides to the medical literature (editorial). JAMA. 1993;270: 2096–7.
2. Haynes RB, Mukherjee J, Sackett DL, et al. Functional status changes following medical or surgical treatment for cerebral ischemia: results in the EC/IC Bypass Study. JAMA. 1987;257: 2043–6.
3. Duley L, Hnderson-Smart D. Magnesium sulphate versus diazepam for eclampsia (cochrane review). In: The cochrane library, Issue 2. Chichester: John Wiley & Sons, Ltd.; 2004.
4. Lau J, Antman EM, Jimenez-Silva J, Kupelnick B, Mosteller F, Chalmers TC. Cumulative meta-analysis of therapeutic trials for myocardial infarction. N Engl J Med. 1992;327(4): 248–54.
5. Anderson GL, Limacher M, Assaf AR, Bassford T, Beresford SA, Women's Health Initiative Steering Committee, et al. Effects of conjugated equine estrogen in postmenopausal women with hysterectomy: the Women's Health Initiative randomised controlled trial. JAMA. 2004; 291(14):1701–12.

Further Reading

Guyatt G, Rennie D, Editors. User's guides to the medical literature: a manual for evidence-based clinical practice. Chicago: AMA Press; 2002. (www.ama-assn.org).
Guyatt GH, DiCenso A, Farewell V, Willan A, Griffith L. Randomized trials versus observational studies in adolescent pregnancy prevention. J Clin Epidemiol. 2000;53:167–74.
Haynes RB, Sackett RB, Gray JMA, Cook DC, Guyatt GH. Transferring evidence from research into practice, 1. The role of clinical care research evidence in clinical decisions. ACP J Club. 1996;125:A14–5.
Muir Gray FA, Haynes RB, Sackett DL, Cook DJ, Guyatt GH. Transferring evidence from research into practice, III. Developing evidence-based clinical policy. ACP J Club. 1997;126:A14.
Oxman AD, Sackett DL, Guyatt GH, for the Evidence-based Medicine Working Group. Users' guides to the medical literature, I: how to get started. JAMA. 1993;270:2093–5.
Richardson WS, Wilson MC, Nishikawa J, Hayward RSA. The well-built clinical question: a key to evidence-based decisions. ACP J Club. 1995;123:A-12.

Chapter 2
Formulating a Focused Clinical Question

It is important to articulate your need for information into a well-formulated clinical question. The question serves as a starting point for literature search and hence must have a degree of focus that strikes a balance between getting too many 'irrelevant' articles and 'not getting any article at all'. Experts often distinguish between 'focused' questions and 'general' questions. Focused questions specify the type of patients, intervention under consideration, comparison and outcome. General questions usually start with 'what', 'where' and 'how'. For example, what is 'SARS'? What is the pathology of acute myocardial infarction? How do bacteria enter brain? Where does malaria occur? Some authors like the term 'background' questions for general questions (and hence foreground for focused questions). These terms mysticise, and hence, I do not favour them.

Components of a Focused Clinical Question

The components of a clinical question are often described using the acronym 'PICO', where

- P = Patients or population or problem
- I = Intervention
- C = Comparison
- O = Outcome

Let us elaborate them.

- P: 'P' may refer to type of patients. You may specify age, sex, race, disease severity and co-morbidity, which should be similar to the patients under consideration or to the type of patients of interest to you. Sometimes, a question arises: Does P stand for patients, population or problem? My answer is all of them. A complete description is 'population of patients with a problem'. Problem refers to the disease condition. The word 'population' comes here because EBM is based on

K. Prasad, *Fundamentals of Evidence-Based Medicine*,
DOI 10.1007/978-81-322-0831-0_2, © Springer India 2013

evidence from research. Research typically studies a sample of patients but always attempts to infer about the population of patients represented in the sample. Sometimes, you may only refer to the problem. For example, in the question, 'In rheumatoid arthritis, is methotrexate more effective in inducing long-term remission than chloroquine?', only problem (condition or disease) is mentioned.

- I: 'I' stands for 'intervention' of interest – usually the new intervention. This applies to a treatment question. In case of diagnostic test question, 'I' stands for 'index test'. This means the test which is of interest to you. The most versatile expanded term for 'I' is 'independent' or 'input' variable. In treatment question, the input variable is the 'intervention'. In diagnostic test question, it is the 'index test'; in prognosis question, it is the prognostic variable; and in harm question, it is the exposure to potentially harmful agent. Thus, 'independent' or 'input' variable covers all of these. Some experts expand 'I' to 'indicator'. An indicator variable may indicate the likely prognosis or diagnosis and thus covers a prognostic variable or index test.
- C: 'C' stands for 'comparator' or 'comparison' or 'control'. I prefer the term 'comparator' because 'comparison' to some readers means both the interventions and tests – one versus another. Actually only one intervention to which the new intervention is compared comes under this letter.

  In case of diagnostic test, the comparator is always a 'gold standard', which correctly labels (classifies) 'disease present' or 'disease absent' with perfect accuracy.
- O: 'O' stands for 'outcome'. The word 'outcome' here refers to health consequences of exposure or intervention. In case of intervention, it refers to 'patient relevant outcomes' like what happens to the patients as a result of treatment. Clinicians usually mean 'mortality and morbidity', but outcome also includes adverse effects related to the intervention. You should also consider both *beneficial* as well as *adverse effects* of the intervention. Outcome in case of diagnostic test is accurate diagnosis of the patient's problem or condition.

Variations of PICO

1. PECO: Here 'E' stands for 'exposure'. In questions about harm, the potentially harmful agent to which the patients or people are exposed will come under 'exposure'. In prognosis question, the prognostic factor may be taken as the 'exposure, even though it may be a demographic characteristic of the patients like age. Questions like 'whether mobile phone use causes brain tumour' is better formulated with '*E*' in P*E*CO than '*I*' in P*I*CO.
2. PIO or PEO: Sometimes, there is no separate 'çomparator'. For example, if all patients are exposed, there is no comparison with unexposed, though comparison may occur across different levels of exposure. If our question is whether age is a prognostic factor for outcome after head injury, we are comparing those with

older age to those with younger age, or vice versa, but all patients have some 'age'. If you do not know which age to compare to which one, it is not possible to separately identify *E* and *C*. Often there is a linear relationship with perceptible change in outcome for every 5-year change in age.

If you are interested in the question of whether blood pressure (BP) is related to vascular events, you may not be able to state which blood pressure to compare to which one? In fact, you may think (and rightly so) that both lower as well as higher BP may be related to increase in vascular events. In such a situation, it is much easier to use the version 'PEO' than 'PECO'.

3. 'PO': Sometimes, the clinical question is very simple. For example, consider a patient who is diagnosed to have amyotrophic lateral sclerosis (ALS). Patient asks: How long will I survive? You don't know and decide to find this from literature. As there is no treatment for this condition, the question may be formulated as follows: What is the length of survival for patients with amyotrophic lateral sclerosis? The question only has 'patients with ALS' and the 'outcome'. Hence, PO is all that is relevant for this question. Another situation where only 'PO' is relevant is when our interest is to describe phenomena, perception or behaviour. For example, 'How do mothers feel about their children in ICU?' This question asks about perception and has only P (children in ICU), and O = mothers' feelings.
4. PICOT or PECOT: Here the added 'T' stands for 'time'. Proponents of PICOT argue that time period of interest over which the outcome of interest occurs needs specification. In the end, all patients and all of us are dead, and hence, any question (of intervention, harm and prognosis) inherently refers to outcome over a period of time. Therefore, this time period (T) needs specification. However, sometimes this is not relevant. For example, in the above question regarding length of survival in patients with ALS, there is no need to specify the time period. The question seeks to know the length of survival in such patients. However, other questions like mortality after thrombolysis in patients with acute myocardial infarction may rightly require specification like 30-day mortality.
5. PICOS: Some experts add 'S' to PICO, where 'S' stands for 'study design'. It prompts the clinicians to specify the most appropriate study design to answer the question. It does help in limiting your search to one publication type. However, for some questions, multiple study designs can be suitable and for all types of questions, systematic reviews/meta-analyses of primary studies based on suitable study design are possible. Thus, it is not useful to specify one type of study design. Thus, PICOS in my opinion is not a very useful acronym.

It is useful to remember the mnemonic PICO/PECO but focus mainly on PIO/PEO, which covers most of the questions we commonly face in clinical practice, where I or E stands for intervention or exposure. Both interventions of interest (say A) as well as control intervention (say B) may be included as 'A' versus 'B' under the letter 'I'. In the end, complete the task by forming an interrogative sentence including all the components of the question.

Types of Questions

Usually, clinicians pose the following five types of questions:

1. Therapy
2. Diagnostic test
3. Prognosis
4. Harm
5. Differential diagnosis

1. *Therapy questions* include all kinds of interventions: medical, surgical, counselling, cognitive behavioural or psychotherapy.
2. *Diagnostic tests* include a single or a combination of strategies (including clinical, laboratory, imaging and others) to differentiate between those with and without the disease under consideration. Screening tests conducted on apparently healthy population may also be included under this, but the characteristics required of a screening test differ from the diagnostic test required to differentiate between patients with one disease under consideration from those with other diseases mimicking the disease under consideration.
3. *Prognosis* questions at the simplest level aim to estimate the future course of patients with certain characteristics, for example, stage I breast cancer. However, the higher-level question may include the following:
   (a) What are the important prognostic factors? Is age (or any other characteristics) a significant prognostic factor?
   (b) Is clinical prediction rule based on a combination of prognostic factors, reliable and valid?
   (c) Is one clinical prediction rule (say X) more accurate compared to another prediction rule (say Y).

In this book, I only focus on the simplest of the question: What is my patient's future course?

4. *Harm* questions address the unfavourable effects of potentially harmful agents (including therapies) on patients.
5. *Differential diagnosis* questions seek to determine the frequency of various disorders in patients with a particular clinical presentation.

Essentially, all questions (except the simplest prognosis question) have patients (the input variable) and outcome variable (see table below). Type of question depends on input and outcome variable (see table below).

Input (independent variable)	Outcome (dependent variable)	Types of question
Therapeutic intervention	Patient – important outcome	Therapy
Diagnostic test (index test)	Diagnosis of the disease (differentiation from mimicking diseases)	Diagnostic test

(continued)

Input (independent variable)	Outcome (dependent variable)	Types of question
Prognostic (indicator) variable which indicates the likely course of the disease	Patient – important outcome	Prognosis
Potentially harmful agent	Adverse effect on patients	Harm
Clinical presentation	Various disorders	Differential prognosis

Specifying a Proper Study Design for the Type of Question

It is useful to keep in mind the objectives of the different question types. There are two kinds of objectives: one to properly label the patients at a time point when you see them (classification) and second to see what happens to patients subsequent to exposure (consequential). The first usually requires one time contact and the study design is cross sectional. Sometimes, to know what the patient had at the time point of interest requires follow-up, but the aim is to know the condition at the specified time point. In the second, we need to know whether the patient had exposure at one time point and what was its consequence (outcome) at second time point. Thus, we attempt to examine exposure–outcome relationship. The study designs for examining exposure–outcome relationship are case–control and cohort studies. As special case of cohort study where a set of patients are allocated to receive the exposure through a process similar to coin tossing (random allocation) is called randomised controlled trails (RCT). A drug, device or surgery may be studied in an RCT for both their benefits and harms. Thus, RCT is the best study design for therapy as well as harm, but patients cannot be allocated to potentially harmful agents by the researcher for ethical and practical reasons, and, therefore, for harm, other study designs like case–control or cohort are the next best. For prognosis, there is a need to follow up patients from exposure to outcome, and hence, cohort design is the most appropriate.

For each study design, one can find systematic reviews or meta-analyses. Thus, your first attempt should be to locate systematic review of the studies of designs appropriate to the type of question.

Examples

Therapy Questions

In the scenario of the stroke patient presented in Chap. 1, the question may be stated as follows:

> 'In patients with acute ischaemic stroke within few days after onset, what are the effects (improvement in functional outcome and bleeding episodes) of I.V. heparin (standard) compared to oral aspirin over six months'.

Template for Therapy Question

In P (patients with a certain disease) what are (O) the effects (beneficial and adverse) of E (new or experimental intervention) as compared to C (control intervention)?

Diagnostic Test Questions

A 50-year-old gentleman with COPD who is bedridden suddenly develops breathlessness and hypertension. You suspect pulmonary embolism and order ventilation–perfusion (V/Q) scan; however, you do not know and want to know how good is V/Q scan in the diagnosis of pulmonary embolism. Before searching the literature, you start to formulate the question:

- Patients: middle-aged men with COPD, bedridden and suspected to have pulmonary embolism
- Index test: ventilation–perfusion scan
- Comparator: gold standard (pulmonary angiography)
- Outcome: diagnosis of pulmonary embolism

Template for Diagnostic Test Question

In (P) patients (middle aged with COPD, bedridden) suspected to have pulmonary embolism (PE), how accurate is I (ventilation–perfusion scan) in diagnosing PE?

Note: There is no need to specify gold standard as 'C' because comparison in all diagnostic tests is with gold standard which gives the correct diagnosis of the condition under consideration; and outcome is accuracy of diagnosis. You have to specify only P and E.

Prognosis

In prognosis, the simplest form of question is: In (P) patients with a disease, how big is the risk of (O) certain outcomes (adverse consequences on health) as was mentioned in earlier section on questions (section "Variations of PICO")? This is a descriptive level question. But on analytic level, one may address the question of relationship between a potential prognostic variable and outcome. The question may take the following form: In (P) patients with intracerebral haemorrhage, does intraventricular extension (E) increase the risk of death (O) in the first week?

Harm

A 55-year-old patient on follow-up for migraine present to you with a newspaper report indicating that mobile phone use may cause brain tumour. He is concerned that he may be at risk of developing brain tumour because he uses mobile phone regularly. You do not know the answer and promise to get back to him after examining the literature. So, what is the clinical question?

P: People who regularly use mobile phones
E: Usage of mobile phone
O: Brain tumour

The template may be as follows:

Is there a risk (if yes, how much) of development of brain tumour (O) in middle-aged person (P) who regularly use mobile phone (E)?

Note: Here, migraine has not been given any reference as the existing knowledge does not suggest that it may have any influence on brain tumour development due to mobile phone use.

Differential Diagnosis

A 60-year-old gentleman presents with recurrent episodes of loss of consciousness over the last 5 years. He has been examined by many doctors, but no diagnosis has been reached. He presents to you for a diagnosis and management. You decide to review the literature for this. What is the clinical question?

The template may be as follows:

In elderly males (P) presenting with recurrent episodes of loss of consciousness (E), what is the frequency of various disorders (O)? likely to cause it.

Usefulness of Formulating a Well-Structured Question

The advantages of formulating a well-built question are:

(i) It helps to focus on the most relevant paper (s).
(ii) It increases efficiency of search for the evidence.
(iii) It helps you to set the desired outcomes, particularly in cases of therapy questions. This is important because many papers address only surrogate outcomes not the clinical (patient important) outcomes.

Chapter 3
Finding the Current Best Evidence

Once your question is well formulated, you need to find the current best evidence to answer the question. To do this efficiently, you may do two things: one, to ask a colleague, and two, to search for evidence. The colleague may guide you to the latest and best evidence or give you some information to facilitate your search. In any case, I think it is good to search some online sources so that you don't miss a recent article. A third source can be the company representatives, who come to inform you of their newer products and claim their (products') superiority or effectiveness. You may ask them to bring reprint of original articles to substantiate their claim.

In any case, an online search is always advisable [1]. A list of information resources for online search is provided below.

Information Resources

Four categories are described [2]:

1. *Studies*: Primary or original studies, for example, those retrieved from MEDLINE/PubMed. More than 20 million articles are indexed in MEDLINE. They need appraisal for clinical application.

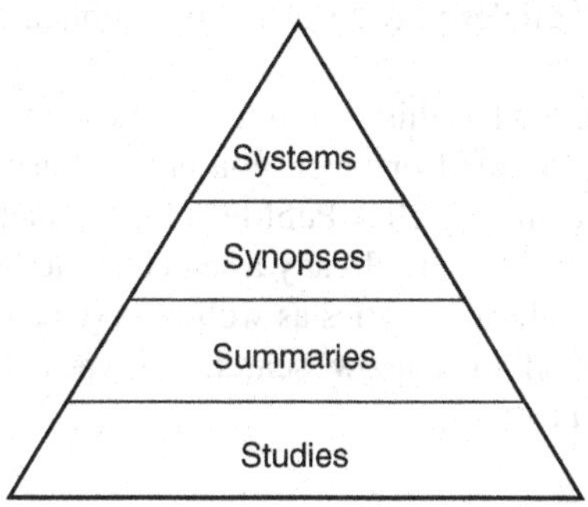

K. Prasad, *Fundamentals of Evidence-Based Medicine*,
DOI 10.1007/978-81-322-0831-0_3, © Springer India 2013

2. *Syntheses or summaries*: For example, Cochrane review which provides systematic reviews of health-care interventions.
3. *Synopses*: There are pre-appraised abstracts published as journals, for example, *ACP Journal Club* or *Evidence-Based Medicine* or *Evidence-Based Nursing*. For a list of pre-appraisal resource journals in various disciplines, refer to www.ebmny.org/journal.html
4. *Systems*: These usually integrate various types of health-care information like clinical evidence, guidelines, primary studies, summaries and synopses. Examples include UpToDate (www.uptodate.com), Clinical Evidence (www.clinicalevidence.com) and Dynamed (https://dynamed.ebscohost.com)

Three search systems, which are free resources, comprehensive and easy to use and list all types of evidence resource, are:

1. Sumsearch
2. TRIP
3. Google (including Google Scholar)

First two are often good resources to begin your search.

Searching the PubMed

PubMed is free and probably the most commonly searched system. The system keeps improving on regular basis and by the time you read this, the system may have added new features. It may be useful to keep in mind:

1. *Simple searching*: Just type in a word, phrase, series of phrases or a sentence in the searching box. Click 'search' and you will get the hits. The choice of word or phrase should be based on your question, probably in PICO format. Order may be any, but often the 'intervention' and 'patients' yield more useful results.
2. *Related articles and reviews*: On the right of the list of articles retrieved, you will find some citations of related articles and below them two options – 'reviews' and 'all related articles'. You may click on them to expand your search. The retrieved articles may be sorted by 'publication date' using the display button.
3. *Clinical queries*: PubMed has this search feature (you may find this on the lower half of homepage of PubMed or when you enter "PubMed" in 'Google', you may have the option to directly click PubMed clinical queries). Here, you can put a term and click search. There is already a search strategy but into 'clinical queries' which gives you relevant studies as well as systematic reviews on the topic and also option of 'broad' or 'narrow' search and types of articles like 'therapy', 'diagnosis' and 'prognostic'.

4. *Limits*: The option helps you to limit your retrieval in PubMed to publication type (like meta-analysis), age and sex of study subjects, year of publication (like last 5 years), language (like English), etc. The option is available in two ways:
   (i) In direct PubMed search, all these options are displayed on left panel and you may click in as many as you want to limit your search.
   (ii) It is also available as button below the search box.
5. *MeSH terms*: MeSH stands for medical subject heading. This is the controlled vocabulary of MEDLINE. Use of MeSH terms is helpful in retrieving can be missed otherwise. You may click on MeSH terms to add your search terms.
6. *History and combining terms:* 'History' tab is one of the options below the search box. By clicking this, you get a list of the search statements that you have used in your most recent search session. They are numbered. You can combine them by entering the numbers after # and choose option of Boolean operators 'AND' or 'OR'.

Summary

In this chapter, you have learnt various options available in the form of databases, systems, search engines and search strategies. You may start with one system and go on to other options as you proceed. Practice in searching helps you to gain expertise. PubMed is free and has many options, which you may find useful in search for the current best evidence related to your question.

Online Sources

Website addresses according to their cost is given below.

A. *Free*: Many sources are free. A partial list of free sites is given in the Table 3.1.
B. *Low cost*: Sources which are less than $100 per year are given below in Table 3.2. ACP Journal Club and Best Evidence are prefiltered sources. They filter for quality and clinical relevance.
C. *Medium cost*: Sources which are between $100 and $250 per year are given in Table 3.3. Of these, Cochrane Library provides full text of systematic reviews. This is an excellent source, if a review concerning the question is present. Unfortunately, it is still in its infancy, and only a limited number of topics (at present only intervention studies) have been reviewed. It has many ancillary databases and a register of controlled trials.
D. *High cost*: These resources are high cost and preferably consulted in library or institutions. These are as follows (Table 3.4):

Table 3.1 Online health information source free sites

Free medical journals	www.freemedicaljournals.com
Sum search	http://sumsearch.uthscsa.edu/
British Medical Journal	www.bmj.com
MEDLINE:	
PubMed	www.ncbi.nlm.nih.gov/PubMed
Grateful Med	www.medmatrix.org/info/medlinetable.asp
Other source	
Emedicine	www.emedicine.com
Medscape	www.medscape.com/Home/Topics/homepages.html
Medical Matrix	www.medmatrix.org/index.asp
ScHARR Netting the Evidence	www.shef.ac.uk/~scharr/ir/netting/
Medical World Search	www.mwsearch.com
Journal listings	www.nthames-health.tpmde.ac.uk/connect/journals.htm www.pslgroup.com/dg/medjournals.htm
Clinical practice guidelines	www.guidelines.gov www.cma.ca/opgs
Cochrane library	www.cochrane.org (only abstracts are free)
TRIP database	www.tripdatabase.com

Table 3.2 Low-cost sources

Resource	Internet address	Annual cost
ACP Journal Club	www.acponline.org/journals/acpjc/jcmenu.htm	$65
Best Evidence	www.acponline.org/catalog/electronic/best_evidence.htm	$85
Harrison's online	www.harrisonsonline.com	$89

Table 3.3 Medium cost sources

Resource	Internet address	Annual cost
Cochrane Library	www.update-software.com/ cochrane/cochrane-frame.html	$225
Clinical Evidence	www.evidence.org	$115
MD Consult	www.mdconsult.com	$200
Scientific American	www.samed.com	$245 ($159 for online access alone)

Table 3.4 High cost source

Resource	Internet address	Annual cost
Up-to-Date	www.uptodate.com	$495
(For trainees)		
Evidence-based	www.ovid.com/products/clinical/ebmr.cfm	$195
Medicine Reviews (OVID)		$1995

Print Sources

There are several publications (including some text books) in print these days that provide reasonably up-to-date synthesis of evidence. The number of such publications is steadily increasing. A partial list is as follows:

- Clinical Evidence (BMJ Publication): £100
  - For students: £45
- Ball CM, Phillips RS. Evidence based on Call: Acute Medicine. London: Churchill Livingstone. 2001. (http://www.eboncall.co.uk)
- Clinical Evidence. Available from the BMJ Publishing Group (httg://www.clinicalevidence.org/) as a semi-annual text or online.
- Dawes M. Evidence Based Practice: A Primer for Health Care Professionals. Edinburgh: Churchill Livingstone; 1999. Can be purchased on-line at http://www.harcourthealth.com/fcgi-bin/displavpaqe.pl?isbn=0443061262 for U.S. $29.95.
- Feldman W. Evidence Based Paediatrics. Hamilton, Canada: BC Decker; 1999.
- Gerstein HC, Haynes RB (editors). Evidence Based Diabetes Care. Hamilton, Ontario: B. C. Decker, 2001 (includes book and database on CD).
- Moyer V. Evidence Based Paediatrics and Child Health. London, UK: BMJ Books; 2000.

References

1. McKibbon KA, Richardson WS, Walker DC. Finding answers to well built clinical questions. Evid Based Med. 1999;6:164–7.
2. Haynes RB, Wilczynski N, McKibbon KA, et al. Developing optimal search strategies for detecting clinically sound studies in MEDLINE. J Am Med Inform Assoc. 1994;1:447–58.

Further Reading

Greenhalgh T. How to read a paper: the Medline database. BMJ. 1997;315:180–3.

Guyatt G, Rennie D, editors. User's guides to the medical literature: a manual for evidence-based clinical practice. Chicago: AMA Press; 2002. (www.ama-assn.org).

Wilczynski NL, Walker CJ, McKibbon KA, Haynes RB. Assessment of methodologic search filters in MEDLINE. Proc Annu Symp Comput Appl Med Care. 1994;17:601–5.

Chapter 4
Therapy: Fundamental Concepts

Introduction

Health practitioners are rightly interested to know whether a new treatment works, whether it makes any difference. A question may arise: difference in what? The answer is: in the outcome of his case or the prognosis of his patient. But there is a problem. The problem is that there are many factors which influence the outcome in a given patient. Some such factors are called prognostic factors, like age, sex, nature of the disease, disease severity, and co-morbidities. The other factors are biases and chance. If we can eliminate these factors and other treatments as the possible cause of a particular outcome, then we can be sure that the new treatment given to the patient has caused the outcome – whether beneficial or adverse. But it is impossible to eliminate the role of these factors. Hence it is difficult, if not impossible, to know for sure whether a given treatment makes a difference in the outcome. Researchers use several strategies to control these extraneous factors; one of which is to use a control group.

Need for a Control Group

Give the treatment to a group of patients and observe the outcome. This strategy is the one most commonly used. But it has its own problems. *First*, the disease may be self-remitting in some or all patients. Thus, whether the patients recovered due to the treatment or on their own, you cannot say. *Second*, there is something called Hawthorne effect – that is, there is a change in response or behaviours of people when they are kept under observation. *Third*, there is placebo effect – that is, patients feel improvement even if something inactive (placebo) is given. If there is a control group who receives the same attention as the experimental one and also receive a placebo, then the Hawthorne and placebo effects cancel out in the comparison between the experimental and control group. For example, studies in early eighties

K. Prasad, *Fundamentals of Evidence-Based Medicine*,
DOI 10.1007/978-81-322-0831-0_4, © Springer India 2013

with a single group of patients reported moderate to marked improvement with thyrotrophin releasing hormone in motor neurone disease, but subsequent controlled trials did not find any significant improvement. *Fourth*, there is something called 'regression to the mean'. To understand this, let us consider a group of healthy subjects with a true mean systolic blood pressure (SBP) of 135 mmHg. They were attending your outpatient department (OPD). As you know, there is physiological fluctuation in SBP and it rises particularly when the patients are being examined by a health-care worker (so called white-coat hypertension). Suppose, if you did not know this and you wanted to test the effects of a new anti-hypertensive drug. You picked up some of the above patients with SBP above 140 mmHg in the OPD. You administered the drug to all such patients. After 1 h you checked their SBP again. Prior to treatment, mean of their SBP was 142 mm, but it came down to 137 after 1 h, and the difference turned out to be statistically significant. Does it mean the drug is effective? The answer is we don't know. The SBP may have come down in normal course without treatment. The reason is that you picked up those with the upswing in their SBP. Such upswings are known to be normal. What happens after the upswings – SBP will come down towards its mean. This phenomenon is called 'regression to the mean'. This happens spontaneously. So, you won't know whether the drug did something or SBP came down because of 'regression to the mean' phenomenon. Patients selected because of high value of any characteristic can be expected to have lower value on subsequent measurements, purely because of phenomenon of 'regression to the mean'.

Randomisation

Randomisation is a method to allocate individual patients or persons who have been accepted for a study into one of the groups (called arms) of a study. Usually, there are two arms: One arm is called experimental or treatment arm and the other is called control arm. Another term for randomisation is random allocation. This should not be confused with random selection, in which the investigator uses a process to recruit sample for the study. This is used to select a representative sample from the study population, usually in a survey.

Randomisation process is like tossing a coin to allocate the patients into the different arms of the study. Let us say there are two arms in a study. Mr. X is a patient who is eligible and has given consent. Now a decision has to be made to put him into either experimental or control arm of the study. You first set a rule that each time a patient is accepted into the study, you will toss a coin – if it comes head, he will go to (say) experimental arm; however, if it comes tail, he will go to control arm. Accordingly, Mr. X comes, you toss a coin – it comes tail; therefore, Mr. X goes to control arm. Likewise, whenever a patient comes, the same steps and rules are followed. Finally, you will have two groups totally created by tossing a coin. As you can imagine, if there are two hundred subjects, approximately 100 will be in experimental arm and another approximately 100 in control arm. Thus, you will have two groups created through randomisation.

The question is why do we randomise? We randomise to create two prognostically similar groups. In the 200 subjects we had, if there were 50 females, you will find roughly (not exactly) half in each group; if there were forty old people, you will find roughly half in each group; if you had 80 diabetics, you will find roughly half of them in each group. It happens because each patient has equal (50–50) probability of going into one of the two arms. This divides all the characteristics, measured or non-measured, visible or invisible and known or unknown, approximately equally into the two arms, provided you have enough number (say hundreds) of patients. When is the number enough? The exact number depends on how many factors you want to balance. Of course, it will be roughly half and half, not exactly. In fact, if you are very unlucky and have small numbers, you might find one-third in one group and two-thirds in another group. This is why you need to check whether the randomisation worked well in your study or not.

There are two more advantages of randomisation – one, you cannot consciously or subconsciously introduce bias in selection of the patients. If you were relying on alternate patients going to one or the other arm – say, medical versus surgical – you may select only the low-risk patients into surgical and the high-risk cases into medical. This is possible if you are deciding the eligibility and taking consent from the patients and you also know that next patient goes to one particular arm (more details on this in Chap. 4). Second advantage of randomisation is that it meets the assumption of all the statistical tests used to compare the two groups.

Intention-to-Treat Analysis

In our hospital in India, serious patients with spontaneous supratentorial intracerebral haemorrhage (SSIH) were all admitted in neurology and treated medically with hyperventilation, mannitol, control of hypertension, etc. Our policy was to treat such patients medically. Our chief of neurosciences, a neurosurgeon, returned after visiting some neurocentres in the UK and USA and convened a meeting of neurologists. The discussion was on the following lines:

Neurosurgeon (NS): I found in all the centres I visited that their policy is to admit all serious patients with SSIH to neurosurgery, particularly those with altered consciousness. Right from the emergency, neurosurgery is involved. Most, but not all, patients are operated upon. My impression is that this approach yields better outcome.

Neurologist (N): I do not believe that surgery has a role in SSIH. I have looked at the available evidence from randomised studies. It does not favour a policy to treat such patients in neurosurgery.

NS: OK, I understand your point. See, your intention is to continue the present policy – that is, all patients are admitted and cared for by neurology service – some of them may require surgery at a later date. My intention is to treat all patients with altered consciousness in neurosurgery so that such patients get early surgery. Let us compare the two policies in a randomised study, particularly for patients with altered consciousness: intention to treat medically with later surgery if required versus intention to treat with surgery early.

N: What will you do with the conclusions?

NS: If the policy of intention to do early surgery is associated with decreased mortality, we will adopt this policy so that right from emergency, patients will go to neurosurgery. Otherwise, the present policy will continue. My impression is that early surgery policy will reduce mortality rate of such patients in our hospital and this will have national or even international impact as regards treatment of such patients.

A randomised study was carried out with 200 patients. 100 patients of SSIH with altered consciousness were randomised to enter neurology and 100 to enter neurosurgery right from emergency. It turns out that 10 patients in the surgery arm died before surgery could be arranged, and 10 died after surgery. In the medical arm, 20 patients died in total.

The question is how to analyse the data – mainly how to analyse the deaths prior to surgery in the neurosurgery arm? If we ignore them, surgery looks better because 20 % died in medical and 10 % in surgical. If we include them in medical arm, surgery looks much better – 30/110 deaths in medical and 10/90 in surgical. If we count them as death in surgical arm, both medical and surgical arm looks similar – 20 % death in each arm.

The answer has to do with what will happen with the conclusions. If we conclude surgery is better, then all such patients will go to neurosurgery right from emergency (a new policy). If the study represents what normally happens, 10 % (or more) are likely to die before surgery, whereas 10 % will die after surgery. The mortality will be 20 %. Even with the present policy, the mortality is the same. Thus, the outcome for the hospital will remain the same but with a costly approach of surgery in at least 90 % of patients. In other words, the conclusion was falsely positive in favour of surgery. If we want to know what results to expect with change of policy from medical to surgical, then everything, which happens after randomisation to an arm, must be counted on that arm. The deaths occurring before surgery have to be counted in the surgical arm because this is what is likely to happen in real settings. Thus, the medical arm will have 20 % mortality and so will the surgical arm.

An analysis which counts all outcomes pertaining to an arm in a randomised trial in that arm only irrespective of whether the patients receive the intervention or not is called an 'analysis based on intention-to-treat principle'.

What Does It Tell Us?

It tells us what outcomes to expect with one policy versus another. It tells us what happens with a policy under real (usual) circumstances. In other words, what does happen or what does an intervention do? This is often different from what can an intervention do. (Please see below).

Another Example

A new drug to reduce cholesterol came into being. A study to assess the effectiveness and safety of the new drug randomised 1,103 patients to the treatment arm and 2,789 to placebo arm [1]. In the treatment arm, 746 patients complied to the protocol (treatment), of which 112 (15 %) died, whereas in the placebo group 585 (20.9 %) died, a statistically significant difference (*P* value = 0.0003). Analysed in this way, you may conclude that the treatment is effective in reducing mortality. However, this is a biased analysis. You have taken all patients in the placebo arm and only compliant ones in the treatment arm. In placebo arm also, there were compliants and non-compliants. The compliants in the placebo arm also had only 15.1 % mortality, practically no difference from those in the treatment arm. If you compare compliant patients only in both the treatment and placebo arm, there is no difference. If you compare all patients in the treatment (mortality 20 %) versus all patients in the placebo arm (mortality 20.9 %), there is practically no difference (*P* value = 0.55). This last analysis is called 'intention-to-treat' analysis.

The question is which of the above analysis is likely to be unbiased. Here you have to remember why, in the first place, you chose a randomised design. You did so because randomisation tends to balance the prognostic factors between the two arms on an average. Having done it, you must take its advantage. The only analysis which allows you to take the full advantage of randomisation is intention-to-treat analysis, that is, *attributing all patients (and their outcomes) to the arm to which they were randomised, irrespective of whether they actually received their assigned treatment or not.*

Why Intention-to-Treat Analysis?

If you analyse only the compliant patients, you are likely to get biased results. Why? The reason is that the compliant patients in the two arms may not be prognostically balanced.

You would mix up the effects of treatment and bias introduced by prognostic imbalance. Even if you show balance in known prognostic factors, there is no guarantee that unknown prognostic factors will be balanced. Therefore, the only analysis, which takes full advantage of a successful randomisation, is the one based on intention-to-treat principle. If you don't, you may lose the benefits of randomisation and also the strength of a randomised design. Some experts say you convert a randomised study to a cohort one.

Principle of Intention to Treat (True ITT Analysis) Versus Intention-to-Treat Analysis (Quasi-ITT)

Guyatt and his group distinguish between the principle of intention to treat and the common usage of the term intention-to-treat analysis [2]. The principle of ITT requires that all patients randomised must be included in the analysis in their respective arms. On the other hand, the common usage of the term 'ITT' includes violations of the principle, which means withdrawing patients, after randomisation. There are three usual reasons for withdrawal:

(i) Mistaken eligibility
(ii) Non-compliance
(iii) Losses to follow-up

(i) *Mistaken eligibility*: Consider a trial of steroids in acute bacterial meningitis, in which some cases of viral (aseptic) meningitis are also included inadvertently. Withdrawing the latter may not threaten validity greatly, except if they had adverse effects of steroids. As such outcome of aseptic meningitis is universally good, and hence prognostically the withdrawn groups are likely to be balanced. No major threat to validity arises as the prognostic balance is not disturbed.

(ii) *Non-compliance*: Non-compliance to the treatment to which the patients are randomised arises usually due to the following reasons:

   (a) Adverse effects: more often in experimental treatment group than placebo.
   (b) Perceived lack of efficacy: if the treatment is ineffective and patient is deteriorating.
   (c) Negligent behaviour of the patients: this is likely to be distributed equally in both the groups.

   It is evident that the non-compliance due to (a) and (b) reflects on the risk–benefit profile of the new treatment and hence should not be neglected. In fact, this in itself can be one of the important outcomes to be analysed. Removing the non-compliant patients may in fact paint a rather unduly favourable picture of the new treatment.

(iii) *Losses to follow-up*: This will be discussed under adequate follow-up in the next chapter.

From the above it is clear that non-compliant patients need to be included in the analysis and there should (ideally) be no losses to follow-up. All patients need to be included in the respective arms in the final analysis.

Limitations of ITT

You might have noticed that there are some problems in the concept of ITT. The benefit (and adverse effects) of the treatment can be experienced only by those who take it. If only 50 % of the patients comply with the treatment and all patients are counted in the analysis, then there is bound to be dilution of the effects, both beneficial and adverse, of the treatment. This will result in underestimation of the effects (sometimes, with two active treatments under comparison, there can be overestimation of the effects). Yes, this is right. ITT commonly results in underestimation of effects.

Is there a way to resolve this problem? Some experts think that analysing only the compliers (per-protocol analysis) can solve this problem. This is not right. Compliers in the two groups may not be similar. In the control group, moderately sick may leave the study to seek other treatments, while in the treatment group, such patients may benefit and therefore remain compliant, while some may develop adverse effects and leave. Thus, the kind of patients in the two groups remaining compliant would differ in prognosis. Thus, per-protocol analysis will give biased results. Experts are still working on methods, which will give the estimate of effects of treatment with 100 % compliance.

Note: Most drug controlling agencies (like FDA of USA) insist on ITT analysis for approving new drugs. The reason must be obvious to you. ITT analysis protects against biased results. This is also the reason why editors insist on ITT analysis for publishing a paper.

Concepts Related to *P* Value

P value is meant to answer the question: Are the observed results real or by chance?

We as clinicians might think it may be impossible to determine whether any observation is real or by chance. We are right to some extent, but our statistician 'gurus' have worked out since 1920s a number of (literally hundreds) formulae to suit all kinds of observations. Prior to applying the formulae, they start with a hypothesis which assumes that treatment has no effect (or there is no difference between the two groups). This is called 'null hypothesis'. This strategy may remind you of the widely held assumptions in many criminal justice systems that a person is innocent unless proved otherwise'.

Next step is to check under the above assumption of no effect or no difference – what is the probability of obtaining a result equal to (or more extreme than) what was actually observed in the study? There are many steps in the calculation, but you need not worry about that. If this probability is very small, conventionally taken as 5 % (0.05), then a decision is taken to reject the null hypothesis and consider that the treatment has some real effect or it makes a difference. This 5 % is what is called *P* value (*P* stands for 'probability'). *P* value of 0.05 suggests that the observed result is unlikely to be due to chance, likely to be real.

P (Probability)-value is the probability that the difference observed could have occurred by chance, if the groups were really not different (i.e. under null hypothesis).

In most biomedical and epidemiologic work, a study result where probability value (*P* value) is less than 5 % ($P<0.05$) is considered sufficiently unlikely to have occurred by chance to justify the designation 'statistically significant'.

This raises three questions: (1) Why is it necessary to start with null hypothesis? (2) Why 0.05 (or 5 %) is the cut-off value? (3) How do we calculate P value?

Why is it necessary to start with null hypothesis? (Learning point 1)

A detailed discussion of these questions is beyond the scope of this book, but a few lines are in order. First of all, let me say, you need not always start with null hypothesis. You may start with any hypothesis like the treatment makes a difference of 5 or 10 or 20 % and the like. The problem is as follows: Accordingly your question changes and calculation will have to change, for example, you are asking: Assuming that the treatment makes a difference of 5 %, what is the probability of obtaining a result equal to (or more extreme) than what was observed in the study?

Three problems arise:

1. There is no way to decide what should be your starting hypothesis – may be 5 %, why not 10, 15 %, etc. You may have to change the hypothesis and recalculate as many times.
2. The calculation under 'null hypothesis' is the easiest, whereas it gets tougher with any other hypothesis.
3. The computer packages are set to test only the null hypothesis, which is also accepted worldwide. It will take you several days to calculate on your own.

You would agree that it is better to stick to null hypothesis that tests whether the effect is different from zero.

You know that physicians often use such strategies and arguments. You see a patient with fever in an endemic zone of malaria. The patient has sore throat, bodyache and palpable spleen. You may think this is viral fever (not malaria – the null hypothesis), but you order peripheral smear for malarial parasite. If it turns out to be positive, you reject your null hypothesis, start treatment for malaria even though there is a small probability that peripheral smear may show malarial parasite in people residing in endemic zones and this patient's fever may, in fact, be viral fever. You consider that fever, splenomegaly and positive smear for malarial parasite may all be present by chance in such a small number of cases with viral fever that you reject the null hypothesis. The same strategy is used in statistical tests as described above.

Why 5 % is the cut-off value? (Learning point 2)

Well, this is truly arbitrary, but you may agree that it is reasonable. To understand this, let us conduct a hypothetical experiment.

Five friends A, B, C, D and E gathered to decide who will get a free dinner tonight. Everybody was given a similar coin and asked to toss. They had to stop as soon as they got a 'tail'. Whosoever got the highest number of heads before getting a tail will get a free dinner tonight. Anyone doing a trick will be rejected. A got first head and then tail. B got Head – Head- Head – Tail. C got Head – Head – Tail. D got Head – Head – Head – Head – Tail. Would you believe D or reject him. Many of you might think he was doing some tricks, but some may accept it as just good luck. What about E? He got Head – Head – Head – Head – Head – Tail. How many of you will accept it as good luck and how many will reject him saying he was using some trick. Large majority, if not all, will reject him. But the fact is that according to the law of probability, there is a definite, though small, probability that it all happened by chance. How much is this probability – it is $1/2 \times 1/2 \times 1/2 \times 1/2 \times 1/2 = 0.03$ (3 %). Thus, you see that when the chance (probability) of something happening by chance is as low as 3 %, large majority of you reject him. Based on a similar logic, early statisticians decided that if probability of something happening by chance is <5 %, then they will reject that hypothesis, and consider the result statistically significant.

How do we calculate P value? (Learning point 3)

P value calculation involves one strategy and two steps. The strategy is called 'hypothesis testing' or 'significance testing'. Usually the hypothesis to be tested is called 'null hypothesis' which states, for example, that there is no difference between the IQ of doctors and the general population.

This strategy is similar to what many criminal courts use during a trial of an accused. They start with the notion that 'the accused is innocent until proven guilty'. Then they examine the evidence and arrive at a verdict 'guilty' or 'not guilty'. Similarly, we start with the null hypothesis of no difference and examine the evidence and then either 'reject the null hypothesis' or 'do not reject the null hypothesis'. Rejecting also means 'statistically significant difference'. Not rejecting may not necessarily mean 'no difference'. Sometimes, it may mean that the study was not conducted well or had inadequate sample size. Just as in criminal cases, 'not guilty' may be due to inadequate investigation and evidence.

Examining the evidence essentially means finding the signal-to-noise ratio. If this ratio is high (means signal is much more than noise), then we reject the null hypothesis (that there is no signal). When is the signal large enough to reject the null hypothesis? This is known by comparing the obtained ratio to the known distribution of this ratio under null hypothesis. If the probability of obtaining this ratio under null hypothesis is less than 5 %, you reject the null hypothesis.

The steps involved are (1) from the sample data, calculate a quantity (called a 'statistic') which gives the magnitude of the difference between what is found (observed) in the study and what is expected under null hypothesis. This is the signal. A measure of variability in the population (like standard error) is taken as the noise. The ratio between the two is the signal-to-noise ratio. (2) From a known distribution of the ratio (statistic), find the probability of obtaining a value of the statistic (the ratio) as extreme (or more) as the one actually observed, if the null hypothesis were true. This is the *P* value.

Example: Let us have a hypothesis that the females have a different (higher) IQ than males. How do we statistically approach to reject or accept this hypothesis? We first assume there is no difference (the null hypothesis). Next, we take a representative sample of males and females. We measure their IQ. As you know, all males or all females will not have the same IQ. There will be some variation among them. This variation is like the noise. If there was no variation, we won't need any statistics. We, in fact, could just take one male and one female – measure their IQ and see whether there is any difference or not. But since there is some variation, we need to assess many males and many females – find the mean IQ of males and mean IQ of females. The difference in the means is the signal. Noise is some measure of the variability in the IQ.

We take the ratio of signal to noise. Then, we determine the probability of seeing this big ratio (or more) if there was no difference among males and females. If this probability is small (typically <5 %), then we reject the null hypothesis of no difference and accept the alternative, i.e. the IQ of females is different from those of males. To know whether it is higher or lower, you must look at the means and decide. The signal-to-noise ratio bears different names depending on the type of data. For categorical data, it may be called chi-square (pronounced like kai-square). For numerical data, it may be called 't' or 'F'. Accordingly, the names chi-square test, *t*-test or *F*-test, etc. are used (details are beyond the scope of this book).

Confidence Interval

These days you often see a number of poll results on TV. They say 60 % people approve A as the prime minister or president. Exit poll suggests that such and such party will get 60 % of seats in parliament and so on. If you have watched carefully, they also often present in small letters: error ±3 or ±5 % or any other figure. What does this error mean? This means that their finding of 60 % is based on a survey of certain number of people (called 'sample') and cannot be taken as the truth. If the error is ±3 %, it means the actual approval rating may be as low as 57 % (60−3) or as high as 63 % (60+3). It may be 59 or 61 % or any figure between 57 and 63 %. Another thing to ask is the level of certainty with which they are saying this. I guess, they say with 95 % level of certainty or they are 95 % sure that the actual approval rating of Mr. A is somewhere between 57 and 63 %. This is what is known as 95 % confidence interval (CI). Confident is certain or sure; interval is range. So *confidence interval is the range within which you are sure to a specified (say 95 %) level that the actual (or true) value lies (Learning Point 1).*

The ends of the interval (like 57 and 63 %) are called the limits of the CI, whereas the width of CI refers to the whole extent (in our example, from 57 to 63 %). Why do we need this? Well, we need this because pollsters or researchers do not study the whole population (of voters or patients with a disease). They study a sample of the population and from this they want to guess what is the true figure in the population. The figure they obtain from the sample cannot be taken as the figure for the population, which may be a bit less or a bit more. You may call this 'margin of error'. This needs to be reflected in the presentation of any study (or poll) results.

Let us try to learn from a familiar example (even though not totally appropriate one). A recently married husband is happy to learn that his wife is pregnant and asks his general practitioner (GP): What is the expected date of delivery (EDD)?

GP: As the LMP is 1 March 2004, accordingly the EDD will be 8 December 2004.

Husband: That's good. I work in a city about 1,000 km away, but December is my vacation month. This is our first baby. I want to be with my wife during this delivery. I will be surely here by 7 December. Is this OK?

GP: No, the delivery may take place earlier or later than 8th.

Husband: Is it OK, if I come 1 week earlier?

GP: Well, you can be 60–70 % sure that the delivery takes place within plus/minus 1 week.

Husband: No, doctor, I want to be more sure than 60–70 %.

GP: Well, you may be 95 % sure that the delivery will be within plus-minus 2 weeks.

Husband: If I come 3 weeks earlier and plan to stay 3 weeks later than EDD, can I be 100 % sure that I will be here on the date of delivery.

GP: No, I guess you can be 99 % sure. After all, there are things called prematurity and post-maturity. If you want to be 100 % sure, you will have to leave your job and stay with her till she delivers.

Well, the point this example illustrates is that if you want to be more sure, the time interval of husband's required presence will be larger. Thus, 99 % confidence interval will be wider than 95 % confidence interval, which in turn will be wider than 90 % confidence interval. *Therefore, the width of the interval is directly proportional to the specified level of confidence (Learning Point 2).* The bigger the desired level of confidence, the greater is the width of the interval and less the desired level of confidence, less is the width of the interval.

So, the question is as follows: What level should we use? The researchers most commonly use 95 % confidence interval. You may stick, for all practical purposes, to 95 % confidence interval. All subsequent discussions here on C I refer to 95 % CI.

You may ask: How do they calculate the margin of error? Well, there are hundreds of formulae for this. A formula is selected according to the type of data and parameter one is dealing with. To give you a better insight, I illustrate this with an example of calculation and interpretation.

Suppose you want to know whether most people favour A as the next president of the USA. You take a random sample of 24 people from the population of voters and ask them the question: Do you approve Mr. A. as the next President of the USA? (Let's call it Survey I). Suppose you find that 60 % of them favour Mr. A as the next President of the USA. This 60 % is often called approval rating. Does it mean that the majority of people favour him? Sixty percent would suggest yes, but you are not comfortable in saying so, because you have asked only 24 people. Confidence interval (CI) calculation will make it clear. To calculate 95 % CI around a percentage (say, p) obtained in a survey, the formula is $p \pm 1.96\sqrt{[p(1-p)]/\text{sample size}}$.

Here $p = 60\,\% = 0.6$ (in decimals). Therefore, 95 % CI will be $0.6 \pm 1.96\sqrt{\left[0.6(1-0.6)\right]/24} = 0.6 \pm 1.96 \times 0.1 = 0.6 \pm 0.196$, which is approximately (0.6 ± 0.2), which means ($0.6 - 0.2$)–($0.6 + 0.2$) i.e. 0.4 (40 %)–0.8 (80 %). What does it mean? From your survey you can be 95 % confident that the true approval rating of Mr. A is between 40 and 80 %. If it is 40 or 45 %, majority do not approve him; if it is 65 or 80 %, yes, majority approve him. The width (range) of confidence interval is rather too wide; it is not precise. You should do a study with a bigger sample. If you did the survey with 400 people (let's call this Survey II) and you again found 60 % people approving Mr. A, 95 % CI comes to approximately 55 to 65 %, which is precise enough to permit you to say with 95 % certainty that Mr. A has approval from majority (If it is 65 % it is majority, if it is 55 %, even then it is majority). There are two messages in this example:

1. The confidence interval is calculated from the study data itself and depends on the sample size. The *more the sample size, the less is the width of the CI, and the less the sample size, the more is the width of the CI* (*Learning Point 3*)
2. *The less the width of the CI, the more precise is the answer, and the more the width of the CI, the less precise is the answer (results) (Learning Point 4).* However, irrespective of the width if your conclusion is the same at either limits of the CI, it is precise enough. [In this example, with second survey your conclusion with 55 % as well as 65 % is the same – that is, Mr. A has majority approval – he is likely to win the presidency.] If your conclusion at one limit of CI is different from the other end, then the CI is not precise enough. [In the above example, Survey I did not have precise CI because if truth was 40 %, you will conclude that Mr. A did not have majority approval, whereas if it was 80 %, you will conclude that he did have majority approval – the two conclusions are diametrically different].

How Do We Graphically Represent the CI (Learning Point 5)?

We do this by using a point and a line on either side of the point. The point corresponds to the basic finding from your study (e.g. approval rating of 60 %, in both the surveys) represented by a point on the graph, and the length of the lines on either side corresponds to the confidence intervals. The results from the two surveys in the above example will be represented as follows (Fig. 4.1):

Your basic finding (also called 'observed' finding) is probably the 'best guess' about the truth. Guess in sophisticated language is called 'estimate' and hence the point represents the 'best estimate' from your study and is referred to as the 'point estimate'. So, what is point estimate? It's basically what you found (or observed) in your study and is represented by a point on the graph.

As you can see, there is a vertical line at 50 %. This is because your reference figure to know whether it is majority or not is 50 %, above which you will call it majority. For a different purpose (as illustrated below), the reference line is at a different point on the scale, and the scale is also different.

This type of presentation of confidence intervals is most commonly used in reporting trials or meta-analyses of treatments. In this case, the reference line is

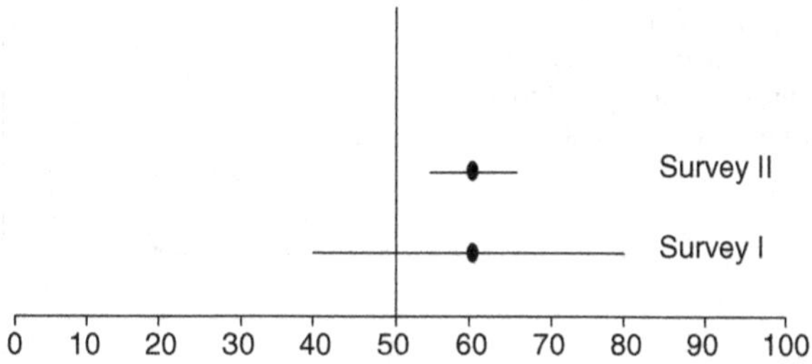

Fig. 4.1 Graphic representation of results from two hypothetical surveys

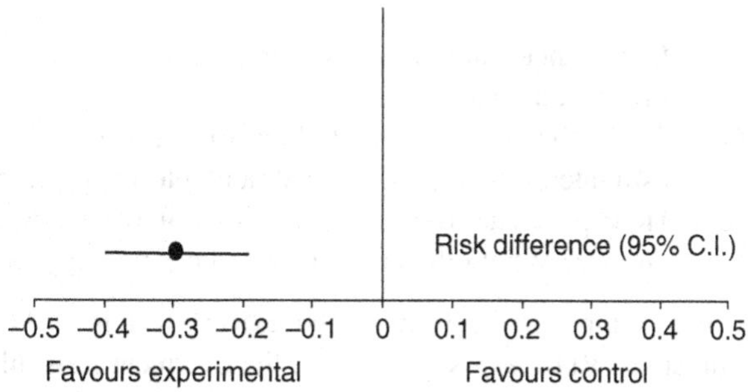

Fig. 4.2 Graphic representation of results from a hypothetical clinical trial

taken as the line of no effect or 'line of null value' or briefly 'null value line'. When there is no effect, the difference between the two treatments will be 'zero', i.e. risk difference will be 'zero'. For example, say the risk of death with experimental treatment is 20 % and with control treatment is also 20 %, i.e. the treatment has no effect and hence the difference is (20 % – 20 %) = 0. However, the risk ratio (relative risk) in this situation is 20 %/20 % = 1. Similarly odds ratio is also '1'. The point is you should carefully see the scale beneath the vertical line and the measure being used – if it is risk difference, the scale at the vertical line will show '0'; if it is risk ratio, it will show '1'. Both are consistent with 'no effect'. Also, with risk difference by convention, the left side of the scale shows minus figures, say –5, –10 %, etc., while right side shows plus figures, like +5 and +10 %. In case of risk ratio, the left side of the scale goes below up to zero, while the right side goes above 1, like 5, 10 and 15.

Let us take a trial with 200 subjects in each arm: 40 (20 %) die in the experimental arm and 100 (50 %) die in the control arm. Fifty percent is 0.5 (in decimals) and 20 % is 0.2. The difference is (0.2 – 0.5) = – 0.3. Ratio is 0.2/0.5 = 0.4. The calculations would roughly yield the following:

- Risk difference (RD) = –0.3 (95 % CI –0.4 to –0.2) (Fig. 4.2)
- Risk ratio (RR) = 0.4 (95 % CI 0.3 to 0.55)
- Odds ratio (OR) = 0.25 (95 % CI 0.15–0.4) (Fig. 4.3)

Figure 4.2 represents the risk difference. The point estimate is 0.3(30 %). The effect of treatment observed in this study indicates 30 % less mortality with the experimental treatment. Ninety-five percent CI covers other effects (parameters) compatible with your study data. Thus, these are three other ways to interpret (or to look at) CI:

Fig. 4.3 Graphic representation of results from a hypothetical clinical trial using ratio measures

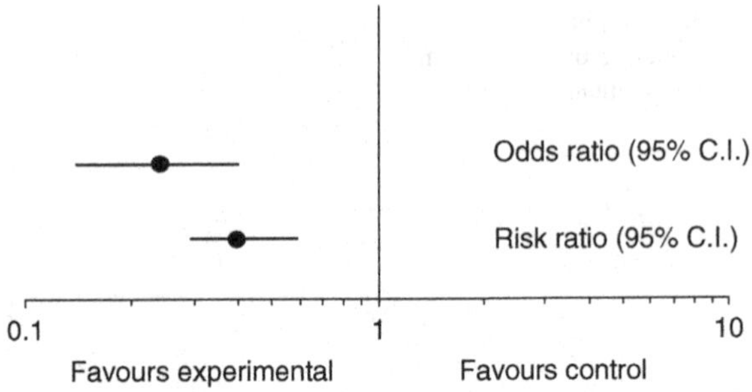

(i) Confidence interval gives you other effects (parameters) compatible with a given study data.
(ii) Given the sample you studied, the most conservative and the most liberal estimate of the effect (of treatment, etc.) is given by the limits of the CI.
(iii) How powerful is the study? Does it have power to give precise enough answer? What effects can be ruled out by the power of the study?

For example, in the example above, RD which is –0.3 (95 % CI –0.4 to –0.2) point estimate of RD=–0.3 suggests that the treatment most likely decreases mortality by 30 % (from 50 to 20 %), but the most conservative estimate with 95 % confidence is that it might decrease by 20 %, and most liberal estimate would be that it might decrease by 40 %, but all figures between 20 and 40 % are compatible with the study data. The study has enough power to say that the true effect of the treatment is more likely between 40 and 20 %. Decreases of >40 or <20 % can be ruled out with 95 % confidence.

Next Question Is: How Do You Interpret CIs from Treatment Studies?

Treatment studies usually compare two treatments – one is called experimental (usually a new treatment) and the other is called control (often, a placebo) treatment.

First, check whether the point estimate is on or very close to the null value line. If yes, then check whether the CI is narrow enough to suggest that there is no difference between the two treatments. If the CI is wide, then you say that the study results do not allow exclusion of an important difference.

If the point estimate is away from the null value, then I suggest two rules to interpret – first is a weak but easy rule; second is a strong (but difficult) rule.

The *weak rule* is that you check whether the CI is crossing the line of null value or not. If it does not cross the line, the study results are conclusively in favour of one treatment over the other. Usually, if the CI is entirely on left of the line of null value, the results conclusively favour the experimental treatment, and if it is entirely on the right of the line, they conclusively favour the control treatment. (If the control treatment is placebo, this would mean that the experimental treatment is worse than placebo, meaning it is harmful, rather than helpful.)

If the CI is crossing the line of null value, then you describe the results as a trend but not conclusive. If the point estimate is on the left of the null value, you report that the results show a trend in favour of experimental treatment but are inconclusive. Similarly for the point estimate on the right of null value line, the results show a trend in favour of the control treatment but are inconclusive. (Sometimes, both the treatments under study are active treatments; accordingly the wording has to be changed.)

The *strong rule* is based on what you would do if the true effect were at one or the other end of the CI. You ask: Would you recommend the experimental treatment if the true effect is at the left end of the CI? Again you ask: Would you recommend the experimental treatment if the true effect was at the right end of the CI? If answer at both ends is the same, then the results are conclusive. If they are different (at one end you will recommend the treatment, at the other you will not), then the results are inconclusive. You can still talk of the trends favouring one treatment or the other (as described in the weak rule).

For example, let us consider a study comparing surgical (say, endarterectomy) versus medical (say, antiplatelets) treatment of carotid stenosis to prevent stroke. Let us say, the surgical treatment is associated with 2 % excess rate of complications (say, perioperative stroke). If the results show that following the perioperative period surgery decreases the stroke risk [risk difference of 4 % (95 % CI −7 to −1 %)], would you consider this a study conclusively in favour of surgery? By the weak rule, yes, because the 95 % CI does not cross the null value line. But let us apply the strong rule. If the true effect of surgery is at −7 %, we will recommend surgery because it decreases the risk of stroke by −7 %, which is much better than +2 % excess risk of stroke associated with the surgery. However, if the true effect is −1 %, we will not recommend surgery because its benefit of −1 % is less than its risk of +2 %. Thus, you see that the recommendations are different at the two ends of the CI. Hence, you conclude that the study was not conclusive or the estimate is not precise. You need more studies to confirm whether the benefit is more than the risk.

Why do I call it a strong rule? Because, it always works and depends on the comparison of clinical benefits versus risk, whereas the weak rule depends only on the statistical calculations. However, the strong rule requires you to think more deeply and asks you to make a judgment whether benefit is worth the risk (and cost). Sometimes, it is difficult to make this judgment.

Relationship Between P Value and Confidence Interval

(What Are the Limitations of *P* Values and Advantages of Confidence Intervals?)

Consider two hypothetical drug trials, placebo controlled: trial A with 10 patients in each arm and trial B with 5,000 patients in each arm. In both the trials, five patients died in each arm. What does it mean – would you say that both trials say the same thing, i.e. the drugs are ineffective? Some of you might say yes. But others would see that trial A cannot say this as strongly as trial B. It is possible that if trial A size is increased to 200 patients in each group, the final tally may be 40 deaths in drug group and 60 deaths in the placebo group – a difference which will be statistically significant ($P = 0.03$) as well as clinically important (NNT = 10). On the other hand, in trial B, even if you increase 200 patients in each arm and the number of deaths increases to 40 and 60 in the drug and placebo arm, respectively, still the

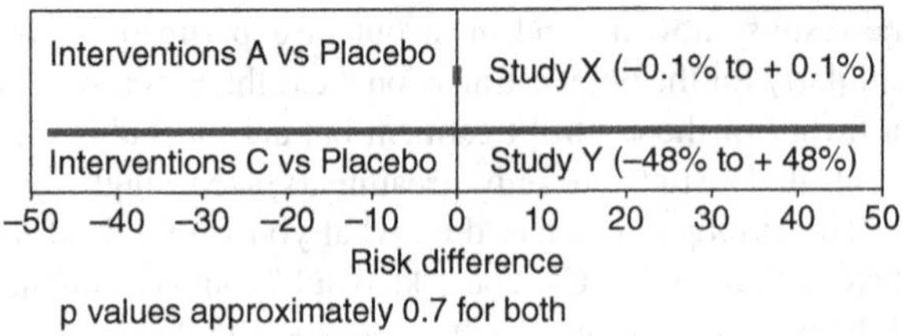

Fig. 4.4 Graphic representation of confidence intervals from two hypothetical trials

difference would be neither statistically significant ($P=0.06$) nor clinically important. In other words, trial B is a case of the 'evidence of absence of benefit' with the drug, whereas trial A is a case of "absence of evidence of benefit". In both instances, *P* values will be close to 1.0. That means *P* value is unable to distinguish between 'absence of evidence of benefit' and 'evidence of absence of benefit'. The confidence interval (CI) does it. Ninety-five percent CI in trial A ranges from – 0.48 to+0.48, suggesting that the study is inconclusive and the data is consistent with –48 % decrease in mortality (benefit) or+48 % increase in mortality (harm). The 95 % CI in trial B ranges from –0.12 % to+0.12 % (both very small figures), suggesting that the treatment is ineffective, neither beneficial nor harmful. This illustrates one of the limitations of *P* value.

Learning point 1:

P value may not distinguish between absence of evidence of benefit and evidence of absence of benefit, but CI does it (Fig. 4.4).

The second limitation can be understood with the following example. Consider two hypothetical placebo controlled two arm trials: trial A with 200 patients in each arm and trial B with 2,000 patients in each arm. In trial A, 40 patients (20 %) died in drug arm and 60 (30 %) in placebo arm, a risk difference of –10 % (*P* equals 0.03). In trial B, 38 (1.9 %) died in the drug arm and 60 (3 %) died in the placebo arm, a difference of –1.1 % (*P* again equals 0.03). You can see that the two results are not the same, yet the *P* values are the same. This illustrates the second limitation of *P* value.

Learning point 2:

A small effect in a study with large sample size can have the same *P* value as a large effect in a small study. *P* value may not be able to distinguish between the two situations (Fig. 4.5).

Let us look at the confidence intervals calculated from the above data. Trial A has 95 % CI=–10±9 %, i.e. from –1 to –19 %. Trial B has 95 % CI from –0.1 to –2 % suggesting that the effect at best is around 2 % (small effect), whereas according to trial A at best, it may be –19 %, which is a big effect. Ninety-five percent CI clarifies that drug A has moderate effect and may have big effect, whereas drug B has only small effect. *P* value does not distinguish between the two situations.

There are some other situations where *P* value is nonsignificant, but CI suggests conclusive results, and *P* value is significant, but CI indicates more studies are required, but this is beyond the scope of this chapter.

The last point about CI is its relationship to the *P* value. The two are the two sides of the same coin, i.e. closely interrelated. Whenever the 95 % CI crosses the

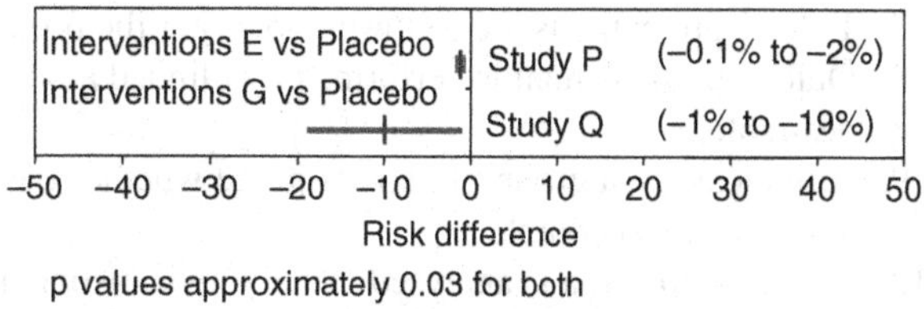

Fig. 4.5 Graphic representation of confidence intervals from two hypothetical trials

line of null value, *P* value is more than 0.05. Whenever it is on one side of the line, *P* value is less than 0.05. Whenever, it just touches the line, $P=0.05$. The smaller it is than 0.05, the more away from the line of null value is the CI. The difference is that CI gives more information than the *P* value. It gives the complete range of possible values of treatment effects compatible with the data, whereas *P* value, even when significant, tells us how far is one of the ends (nearer one) of the CI from the line of null value – nothing more. Thus, CI is particularly useful in determining the precise meaning (precision) of the result and in deciding whether a nonsignificant *P* value means 'absence of evidence' of benefit or 'evidence of absence' of benefit. Many authors often erroneously equate the two. The two situations are not the same. Evidence of absence of benefit means there is enough data (evidence) to say that the benefit due to the intervention is absent, whereas 'absence of evidence of benefit' means enough data (evidence) is not available (or is absent) to make judgment about benefit due to the intervention. This is sometimes expressed as follows: as 'absence of proof (of benefit) is not the proof of absence (of benefit)'.

The Process of Randomised Controlled Trial

An RCT, like any other research, starts with writing a protocol that defines the objectives, research question/hypothesis, eligibility criteria, recruitment procedure, consent outcomes and their measurement and methods of analysis to be used. The actual conduct of the trial goes through the following steps (Fig. 4.1):

1. Eligibility assessment: as soon as a potential subject appears, the investigators assess whether he (the subject) fulfils the eligibility criteria (inclusion and exclusion) of the trial.
2. Consent: if the patient is eligible, he is given all the relevant information in a consent form with opportunity to seek clarification. An informed consent is then taken for participating in the RCT, though the patient has the right to withdraw consent anytime.
3. Randomisation (Random allocation): a patient who is eligible and consenting is then randomly allocated to one of the arms of the RCT.
4. Baseline assessment: all patients are assessed at baseline (before initiating intervention) according to the protocol. Sometimes, it may already be complete at step 1 (eligibility assessment).
5. Initiation of interventions: patients receive the intervention according to the random allocation, either experimental intervention or control.
6. Standard case: all patients receive the standard care.

7. Follow-up: patients are followed up as per the protocol.
8. Outcome assessment is performed by blinded assessors whenever possible and desirable.
9. Adjudication: a group of experts judge whether the outcome measurement are correct and acceptable.
10. Analysis: the data is analysed usually by statisticians.

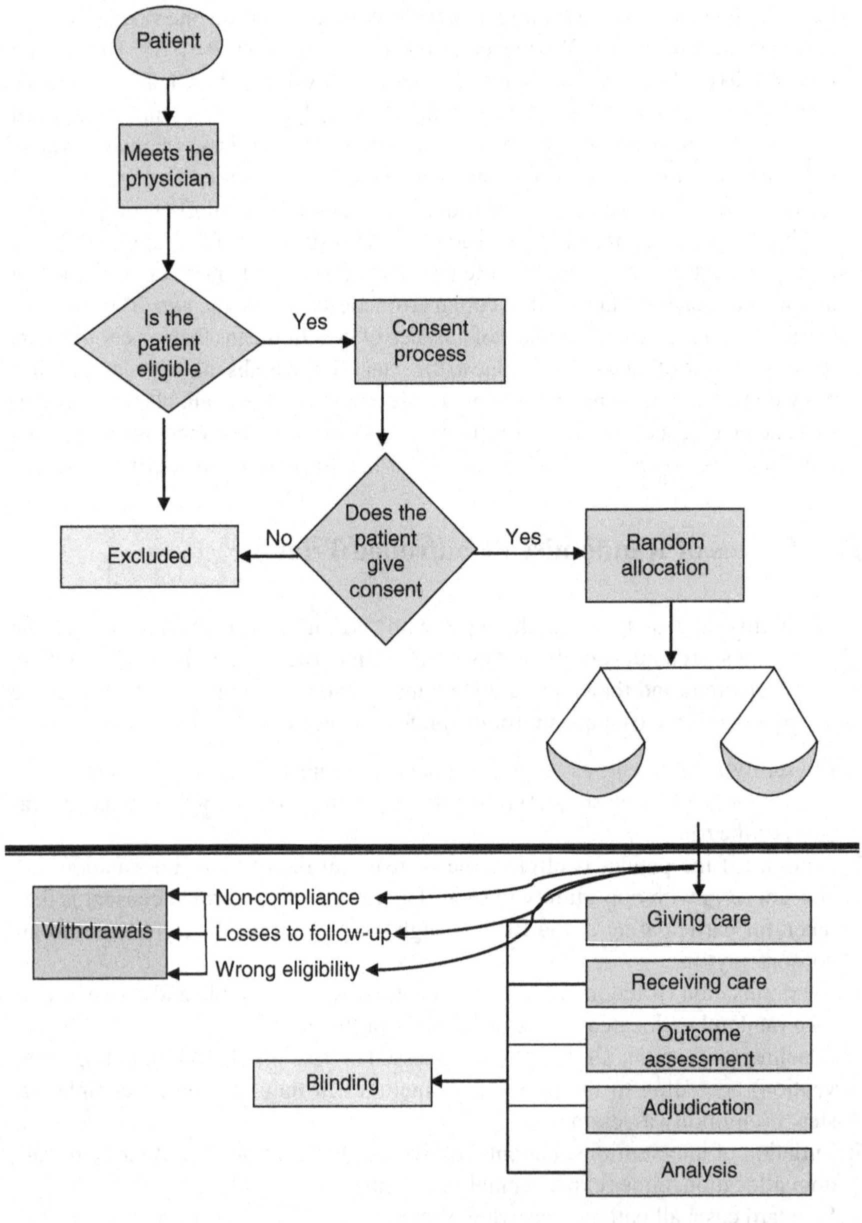

Reference

1. Coronary Drug Project Research Group. Influence of adherence treatment and response of cholesterol on mortality in the coronary drug project. N Engl J Med. 1980;303:1038–41.
2. Fergusson D, Aaron SD, Guyatt G, Hebert P. Post-randomisation exclusions: the intention to treat principle and excluding patients from analysis. BMJ 2002;325(7365):652–654.

Further Reading

Altman DG, Gore SM, Gardner MJ, Pocock SJ. Statistical guidelines for contributors to medical journals. In: Gardner MJ, Altman DG, editors. Statistics with confidence. Confidence intervals and statistical guidelines. London: Br Med J; 1989. p. 83–100.

Chalmers TC, Celano P, Sacks HS, Smith Jr H. Bias in treatment assignment in controlled clinical trials. N Engl J Med. 1983;309:1358–61.

Colditz GA, Miller JN, Mosteller F. How study design affects outcomes in comparisons of therapy, I: medical. Stat Med. 1989;8:441–54.

Coronary Drug Project Research Group. Influence of adherence treatment and response of cholesterol on mortality in the Coronary Drug Project. N Engl J Med. 1980;303:1038–41.

Guyatt G, Rennie D, editors. User's guides to the medical literature: a manual for evidence-based clinical practice. Chicago: AMA Press; 2002. (www.ama-assn.org).

Kunz R, Oxman AD. The unpredictability paradox: review of empirical comparisons of randomised and non-randomised clinical trials. BMJ. 1998;317:1185–90.

Sacks H, Chalmers TC, Smith Jr H. Randomized versus historical controls for clinical trials. Am J Med. 1982;72:233–40.

Sacks HS, Chalmers TC, Smith Jr H. Sensitivity and specificity of clinical trials: randomized v historical controls. Arch Intern Med. 1983;143:753–5.

Yusuf S, Collins R, Peto R. Why do we need some large, simple randomized trials? Stat Med. 1984;3:409–22.

Chapter 5
Therapy: Critical Appraisal: Part 1 (Validity)

Critical Appraisal Questions for a Therapy Paper

Critical appraisal has four main parts:

1. To determine if the study at hand is relevant to your question.
2. To determine if the study is saying the right things (i.e. observed effects are likely to be correct or trustworthy): this is called validity check or quality assessment. In other words, is the information likely to be valid?
3. What is it saying? In other words, what is the potential impact of the treatment? This may be called 'results assessment'.
4. To assess whether the treatment can help you in caring for your patient(s)? I call this applicability assessment, and application to your patient.

So, we have four main assessment tasks:

(i) Relevance assessment
(ii) Validity assessment
(iii) Results assessment
(iv) Applicability assessment and application

Relevance Assessment

Having found the paper, you need to check if it really addresses your question. Check whether the research question in the paper matches your need to an extent that you feel like investing time and effort to go further. Sometimes, the population may not match; at other times, intervention or outcome may not match your need or settings. For example, you wanted to look for the role of surgery in brain haemorrhage, and you found a paper that describes the results of endoscopic neurosurgery in such cases. Your hospital does not have endoscope for neurosurgery and nobody can do it. In this case you may decide to drop this paper and look for some

K. Prasad, *Fundamentals of Evidence-Based Medicine*,
DOI 10.1007/978-81-322-0831-0_5, © Springer India 2013

other paper to deal with your question. Alternatively, you may read only the abstract for getting some information and move to find another paper to proceed with the next steps.

Validity Assessment

Before 1945, researchers were commonly using one group of patients to test any new treatment. Typically, they will use the new treatment in a series of patients and count the outcome (success or failure, death or survival) and compare with their experience in previous series of patients of the same disease.

This method is alright if the treatment effects are 'huge'. Penicillin in pneumococcal pneumonia may be an example. But such treatments are rare these days. Certainly, approval of any new drug for a given condition requires a two-group study (for details, Chap. 3: 'why do we need a control group').

Typically, the investigations are required to have two groups (one experimental and one control), which are similar or balanced in all the factors, that influence the outcome (called 'prognostic factors'). Both the groups receive similar standard treatment, but one group is treated with the new treatment in addition. (The second group is often treated with a matching placebo.)

There are three main questions with regard to validity assessment that is start well, run well and finish well:

(i) Start: Did the authors start with 'balanced' groups?
(ii) Run: Was the initial balance left undisturbed till the end?
In other words, did they maintain the balance during care?
(iii) Finish: Did the study end well? All subjects were followed up; their outcome was assessed properly and analysis was proper.

Let us deal with them individually.

Q.1. Did the Authors Start with 'Balanced' Groups (i.e. at Baseline)?

For this, authors need to *plan* for it, *do* it properly and *check* it.

Here we need to know how balanced groups are formed. The most effective and popular method is similar to 'coin tossing'. We decide that as soon as an eligible patient comes, we will toss a coin – if it comes head, the patient will go to Group A, and if it comes tail, he will go to Group B. If we repeat this process with a 'fair coin and fair tossing', you will find that the two groups do become similar or 'balanced' in all prognostic factors if there are sufficient number of patients. Allocating patients to one group or another in this way is one method of 'random allocation', also called randomisation.

Nowadays, instead of coin tossing, people use a process similar to it, for example, computer 'randomisation'. So, to plan for creating balanced groups requires a plan to randomise. A plan or design to randomise is called 'randomised control design'. Sometimes, a chart is kept ready for randomisation. The chart is prepared using coin tossing or random number tables.

Next, they need to do the randomisation properly. In this context, a problem occurs if the investigator knows the group to which the patient under consideration is going to go. For example, if in a trial of surgical versus medical treatment, the investigator used a chart. If his next patient was to go to surgery and happens to be very sick, he will not include him in the study. He will wait till a 'good risk' case comes. But if he knew that the next patient was to go to the medical group, he will not hesitate to include him in the study. Thus, even though he was using properly designed randomisation chart, his two groups would not turn out to be 'balanced'.

So, it's very important that the group to which the next patient goes is kept undisclosed (or 'concealed') from the investigator who is recruiting the patient. This is best achieved by 'telephone randomisation' or use of similar looking placebos in random sequence with the experimental drug. Someone who is otherwise not involved in the study has the chart or computer, which gives group assignment. The recruiting physician checks eligibility and takes consent. Then he calls the randomising person or centre. After checking that the patient fulfils the key eligibility criteria, the randomising person registers the patient into the study, allots a study number and then assigns the patient to one of the groups. Once registered, the patient irrevocably remains in the study. This process ensures that the recruiting physician cannot anticipate the group to which the next patient goes and thus cannot consciously or subconsciously tamper with the randomisation process. Such a process in which the group assignment of the next patient remains undisclosed (or concealed) from the recruiting physician is termed *'concealed randomisation'*.

Randomisation is called 'concealed' if the group to which the next patient will be assigned remains undisclosed (concealed) from the recruiting physician.

Even after planning (randomised control design) and doing (concealed randomisation) everything properly, we cannot be 100 % sure that the resulting groups are balanced (just as even after careful curriculum planning and flawless teaching, we cannot say that 100 % students will pass). We need to check the results. This means we need to check whether the percentage of patients with the various prognostic factors is similar in the two groups. In other words, are the groups prognostically similar at baseline? This can be done by first recollecting the prognostic factors of the condition and then checking the table of baseline characteristics whether the per cent of patients in the two groups are similar.

Randomisation is no guarantee that the resulting groups will be similar. You need to check the comparability of the groups at baseline.

To summarise, starting well means having a control group, such a control group which is similar to the experimental one (created through randomisation). So, we should check three things:

(i) Is the study design randomised control one?
(ii) Was the randomisation concealed?
(iii) Are the baseline characteristics (prognostic factors) comparable (balanced or similar) between the two groups?

There are three Cs here – (1) control group, (2) concealed randomisation and (3) comparability of groups.

Q.2. Did the Investigators or Subjects Disturb the Balance?

The answer to this question requires checking many things. A story might make it easy to understand. Two housewives, good neighbours and friends, one day went to the market to buy potatoes. Each picked up a box of potatoes, weighing 5 kg. The salesman checked both and each were exactly 5 kg. They came home. While relaxing on sofa and watching TV, they asked the housemaid to bring the potato boxes from the car, wash them and put them back in the respective bags. When the housemaid reported back, she was a bit nervous and asked if she could have a balance. She had found that some potatoes had fallen off from the boxes in the car, but she had done her best to put them in relevant boxes. She wanted to check whether the boxes were of equal weight. She got a balance but had no weights. When she put the two boxes, one on each side of the balance, they were unequal. Assuming that they were exactly equal at the shop, what are the possible reasons for the imbalance now? The possible reasons may arise as follows:

(a) On the way to home – unequal number or size of potatoes may fall off (loss to follow-up).
(b) In the washing process – one group may be washed more thoroughly than the other (unequal care).
(c) Some potatoes may have been mixed up between the boxes (crossovers).
(d) The measuring instrument or process may be biased (measurement bias).

Similarly, in treatment studies, imbalance may arise as a result of unequal care, or crossovers from one group to another or losses to follow-up, or from biased measurement or analysis. So, you need to ask:

1. Were patients in the two groups treated equally? Giving more care to the experimental group with intervention other than the experimental one is called 'co-intervention'.
2. Were the crossovers nil or minimum?
3. Was there adequate compliance?

Again, there are 3 Cs here: co-intervention, crossovers (also called contamination) and compliance (see below for explanation).

Good finish means all patients are followed up (complete follow-up), their outcomes are measured correctly (with reliable and valid instruments and without bias) and the analysis is credible (so that it does not introduce bias).

Again there are three Cs at finish:

- Complete follow-up
- Correct outcome measurement
- Credible analysis

To summarise, the questions to assess therapy paper are related to 3×3 Cs as shown in the Box 5.1:

Let us take each question in detail.

Box 5.1

Start well: 3 Cs

- Control group
- Concealed randomisation
- Comparability of groups at baseline

Run well: 3 Cs

- Co-intervention minimal or nil
- Contamination minimal or nil
- Compliance maximal or adequate

Finish well: 3 Cs

- Complete follow-up
- Correct outcome measurement
- Credible analysis

Q.1. Was There a Control Group?

1A. Why do we ask this question?

We ask this question because improvement may occur in natural course or as a result of Hawthorne effect, placebo effect or regression to the mean.

Many patients improve in a natural course of their disease or remain symptom free. For example, many patients with stroke recover. Many patients with berry aneurysm remain symptom free for a variable length of time. If we do not have a control group, we would not know whether the improvement is due to the new treatment or in natural course.

The control group should be contemporaneous (i.e. current, along with the new treatment group), not historical. The reason is that patients in a previous time period may be prognostically different or may not have had the benefit of organisational or technological advances, which occur with time. Also patients (or people) change their behaviour or perception when they join a research project. This is a natural human tendency. This is known as Hawthorne effect. The effect that we might see in the new treatment group could be due to Hawthorne effect, not necessarily due to the new treatment. But if there is a control group, then any difference, which we observe between the two groups, can be attributed to the new treatment (provided other conditions given below are met) (for placebo effect and regression to the mean, see Chap. 3: Need for a control group).

1B. How do we answer this question?
It would be apparent from the abstract of the paper if there is any comparison with a control group.

1C. How do we interpret the answer?
If the answer is yes, proceed further to evaluate. If it is no, you cannot consider the study as definitive, unless all alternative (competing) explanations for the observed effect can be dismissed. The alternative explanations can be natural history, Hawthorne effect, placebo effect, regression to the mean, effect of a confounder (see below), or co-intervention or bias in outcome measurement.

Q.2. Was Control Group Created Through Random Allocation (Randomisation)? Was Allocation Concealed?

The question has two parts:

First, is there random allocation and second, if yes, is it concealed?

2A. Why do we ask this question?
We ask this question as a follow-up to the first question. If there is a control group, one needs to know whether it is appropriate. How has it been created or assembled? One intuitively appealing method to create a control group is what is called 'matching'. One control matched in certain characteristics to each case is included in the control group. There are two main problems with this approach: First, we need to match for all prognostic factors, then and then only the treatment and control group can be prognostically balanced, and the difference between the two groups can be attributed to the new treatment. Unfortunately, it is very hard, nearly impossible, to find controls matching in all prognostic factors to each case. Even the usual matching of age and sex is so difficult to do that investigators have to accept controls who are 2–5 years younger or older. (Age and sex matched controls are very common for case control studies to determine aetiologic factors. Such studies adjust for other factors in analysis by using multivariate statistics. For treatment studies, this approach is not acceptable.)

Second, matching is possible only for the known prognostic factors. Unfortunately, our knowledge with respect to prognostic factors is very limited. This knowledge is not able to explain, in many diseases, even 50 % of the good and bad outcomes. In other words, there are some known and many unknown prognostic factors. In a treatment study, prognostic factors meet all the epidemiologic criteria of 'confounders' or 'confounding variables' and are often referred to as confounders. You may wonder, if this is the case, how can one balance for unknown prognostic factors? Well, there is a method which can do this, and the method is as simple as coin tossing, but called, in technical language, randomisation (see Chap. 3).

For randomisation to succeed, patient recruitment (or enrolment) into the study should be done without the knowledge of the group (control or treatment) to which the patient will go (be allocated). This is called concealed (or blinded) allocation. The reason is that if the allocation is unconcealed, then those enrolling the patients may systematically recruit sicker – or less sick – patients into one of the study groups. This will either underestimate (if treatment group is sicker) or overestimate (if control group is sicker) the treatment effect, i.e. the study will give a biased result.

Sometimes, there is confusion between 'concealment' and 'blinding' (e.g. of patients and physicians). One way to distinguish between the two is to consider concealment as blinding before initiation of treatment and the usual blinding as blinding after initiation of treatment. Before randomisation, two research steps are necessary – eligibility assessment and consent (See Fig. 4.1). Bias can be introduced in any of these steps.

'Concealed randomisation' is to take place before initiation of treatment, whereas 'blinding' involves steps at and after initiation of treatment.

Consider a trial comparing open versus laparoscopic appendectomy in acute appendicitis. A patient comes who has severe symptoms and signs; the resident knows that the next eligible patient is to go for laparoscopic surgery. He feels that this patient is too sick for laparoscopy and, therefore, declares him 'ineligible'. But when next slot is for open surgery, he does take even the sickest patient. On the other hand, when he finds a less sick patient and the next slot is for laparoscopy, then he considers him eligible. In this way, the open group will have sicker patients than the laparoscopic group and the results of the study will be biased. One can deal with this problem by asking every patient of the condition, who comes to the hospital to be randomised (many would consider this too authoritarian and mechanical, even unethical), but the problem may resurface at the next step that is taking consent. It is a common knowledge that success or failure to obtain consent can be heavily influenced by doctors through the way they explain the potential risks and benefits of participating in a study. The bias can easily be introduced in the same way as in assessing eligibility. There is no way to deal with this problem. Certainly patients cannot be forced to consent for a study.

The following real-life example may illustrate this patient. In 1996, a group of Australian investigators reported a trial of open versus laparoscopic appendectomy in acute appendicitis. Randomisation procedure involved sealed envelopes (containing a paper slip containing an order to do one type of surgery). When an eligible patient came, the resident on call opened the next envelope and the patient went for the surgery indicated on the paper slip inside. Only attending (senior) surgeons were trained for the laparoscopic procedure, whereas all surgeons including residents could do the open surgery. During the day, the trial ran smoothly but during the night, senior surgeons were a bit reluctant to come for the laparoscopic surgery. Residents on night duty developed a practical solution: if an eligible patient came, they held the translucent envelopes up to the light. If the order dictated laparoscopy, they passed over this envelope and went to the next one and so on till they found one that dictated an open procedure, and they opened that envelope and carried out the open surgery. The first eligible patient in the next morning (or day) was then allocated to the laparoscopic group according to the passed-over envelope. If patients who presented in the night were sicker (as they usually are) or the residents had less expertise than the senior surgeons (which is normally expected), the resident's tactics would bias the results against the open procedure.

2B. How do we answer the question?
To do this, read the methods section of the paper. Randomisation is considered concealed if:

(a) There is a proper placebo in random sequence to which those enrolling the patients are blinded
(b) Those enrolling the patients have to make a telephone call to a centre or person who uses a list or computer to assign the patient to one of the arms of the study. Before revealing the allocation, eligibility and consent are verified and the patient is registered into the study. Once registered, the patient remains irrevocably in the study.

A third somewhat less secure approach is to have serially numbered and opaque envelopes, which can be accessed one by one after eligibility and consent is ascertained. The envelope contains the allocation for the patient.

2C. How do we interpret the answer?
If any of the above three methods are used for randomisation, you can conclude that the allocation was concealed.

Randomisation is clearly not concealed if:

(a) A list displaying the allocation is used
(b) Alternate patients are assigned to one arm or the other
(c) Odd or even date of birth is used to assign patients to one or the other arm.

More often, the method of randomisation is not described in sufficient detail to clearly decide about concealment.

Lack of concealment of allocation or unclear description casts doubt about the strength of evidence in the study, but all is not lost. You should move to the next question.

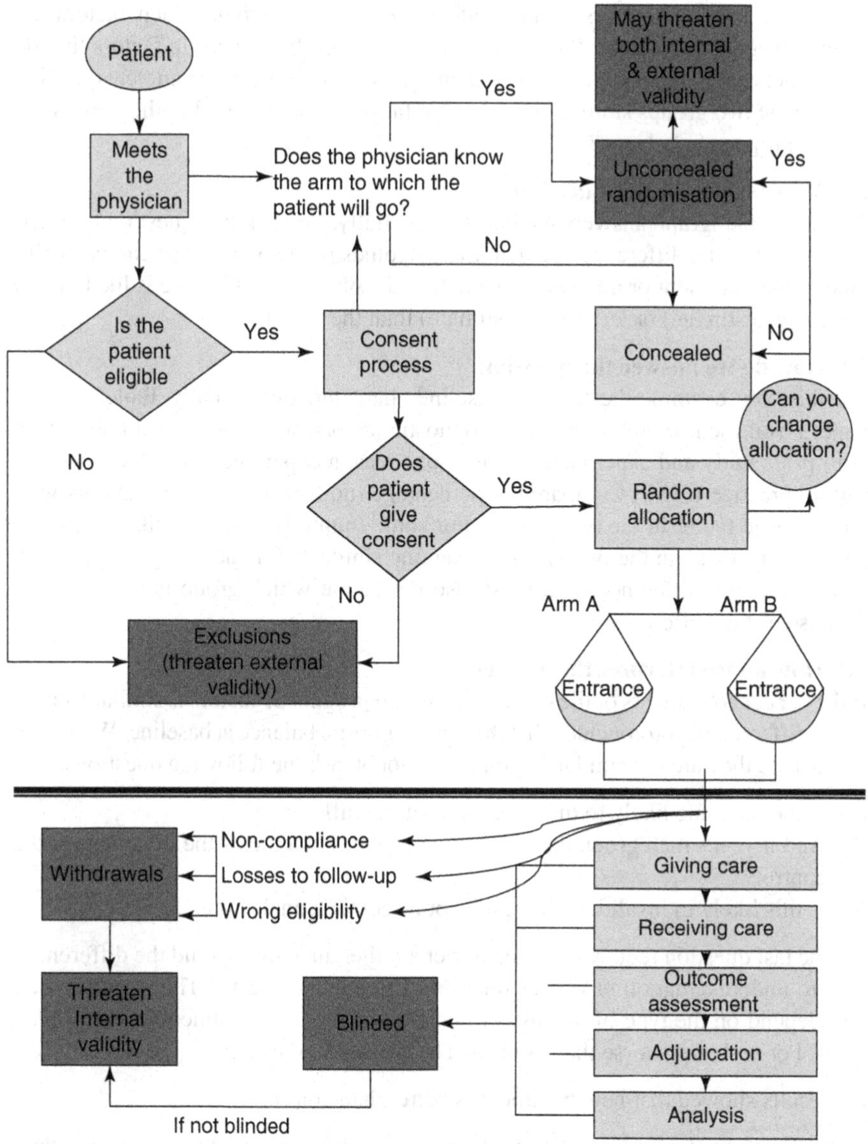

Q.3. Were the Groups Balanced (Comparable or Similar) at Baseline?

This is a very important point to check. You want to know whether the new treatment makes a difference in the outcome, but to know this, there must be no baseline difference between the treatment and the control group. Difference in what?

Difference in those factors, which can influence the outcome. Such factors are called 'prognostic factors'. We need not bother about differences in factors that do not influence the outcome (e.g. sex in meningitis). Therefore, the complete question is, 'Are the two groups similar in prognostic factors at baseline?' In other words, 'Is there a prognostic balance?'

3A. Why do we ask this question?
The above paragraph answers the question partially. You ask this question to determine whether the difference between the outcomes in the two groups can be attributed to the treatment or not and also whether the observed difference is likely to be more (overestimate) or less (underestimate) than the real difference.

3B. How do we answer the question?
For this, you examine the table of baseline characteristics (usually Table 1 of the paper). You focus on the important prognostic factors, which you must know from your prior study and experience. (This is one reason experience/expertise is necessary to practice EBM.) Compare the percentage (not number)[1] of the patients with a prognostic factor in the two groups. For some (numerical) factors like age, compare the mean age in the two groups. Examine similarly for each prognostic factor. If you find any difference, you must also determine which group is at advantage because of this difference.

3C. How do we interpret the answer?
If the per cent of patients or the mean value for all prognostic factors is similar (ignore slight difference), you conclude that there is prognostic balance at baseline. Whenever you decide they are not similar or you are in doubt, ask the following questions:

(a) Is the outcome likely to differ because of the difference?
(b) And if yes, which group is likely to have better outcomes – the treatment or the control?
(c) Is this likely to invalidate the results or affect the conclusions?

The last question requires you to answer another question. Would the differences lead to underestimation or overestimation of treatment effects? The interpretation will depend on the type of results – whether showing new treatment as better than control or no better/worse than control. The two situations are:

I. Results showed that new treatment is better than control:

(i) If the treatment group is at advantage and favoured by the difference, then there will be overestimation of treatment effect and this may compromise the validity of the above results.
(ii) If the treatment group is at disadvantage because of the difference, then there will be underestimation of treatment effect and even then if treatment is

[1]*Number is not important, because they may be very different without much problem. Sometimes by design, investigators keep in the treatment group double the number of patients than the control groups. Obviously, the number of patients for each prognostic factor would be approximately double that in control group, yet the percentage would be the same.*

turning out to be better, you cannot complain. The difference, in fact, strengthens the results and the conclusion.

II. The results show that the new treatment is worse or not better than control:

(i) If the difference puts treatment group at advantage, and yet the results do not favour the group, the results and conclusion are stronger.
(ii) If the difference puts treatment group at disadvantage, then there will be underestimation of treatment effect, and you can question the validity of the results.

You do this exercise for each prognostic factor and if all the differences support the results, then the conclusions are valid. If some favour the results and some disfavour it, you need to check whether authors report an analysis that adjusts for the differences – usually called 'adjusted analysis'. Usually adjusted analysis consists of some form of regression (logistic, Cox or multiple) (details of these are out of the scope of this book). Suffice it to say that if the regression analysis also favours the result, then the prognostic imbalance at baseline probably does not matter much; otherwise, obviously it does.

At the end, you may conclude one of the following:

(i) There is practically no prognostic imbalance at baseline.
(ii) There is prognostic imbalance at baseline, but adjusted analysis supports the conclusions.
(iii) There is prognostic imbalance and no adjusted analysis, but the imbalance does not invalidate the conclusion.
(iv) There is prognostic imbalance and no adjusted analysis. The imbalance compromises the validity of the conclusions.

Q.4. Was There Any Co-intervention Bias?

Co-intervention refers to any intervention other than the ones being studied. After randomisation if patients receive co-interventions unequally in the two groups and if these affect outcomes, they can introduce bias between the groups being compared. This bias is called co-intervention bias.

Having said this, let us remember that most interventions have adverse effects. During the course of a trial if a patient develops an adverse effect, all the necessary treatment has to be offered. If a drug is compared with placebo, the drug arm alone would obviously have adverse effects and also the necessary treatments to deal with the adverse effects. Not surprisingly, then co-interventions would obviously be unequal in the two groups. Usually such co-interventions would only affect the consequences of the adverse effects, and the final outcomes would still tell us the overall effects of the drug.

In any case, if one study arm receives interventions other than usual care and the one being studied, this will be unacceptable. I prefer, therefore, to define co-interventions as any intervention other than usual care and the one being studied.

4A. Why do we ask this question?
In studies, unequal provision of co-intervention may introduce bias in the results. The risk of this happening is less in studies with placebos because care providers are not fully aware of who is receiving what and thus are unlikely to provide unequal care other than the usual.

4B. How do we answer the question?
Results section would describe the kinds of interventions provided to the patients in the two arms. Many studies are silent about this, while others give a table comparing the frequency of use of co-interventions.

4C. How do we interpret the answer?
First consider only those co-interventions, which are likely to influence the outcome. Next, assess whether the differences in the frequency of use would lead to distortion of the estimation (underestimation or overestimation) of the effects. Then consider how the direction and degree of distortion influences the final results.

Q.5. Was There Any Crossover (Contamination)?

Contamination occurs when the control group receives part or all of the new intervention. When the comparison is between two active treatments, contamination occurs when patients in one arm receive the treatment of the other arm.

In comparison between surgical and medical treatment, some patients from medical arm may opt for surgery and vice versa. Such a whole-scale contamination is called 'crossover' (please note this usage of the term 'crossover' has nothing to do with 'crossover trials').

5A. Why do we ask this question?
Contamination tends to blur the difference between the two treatments (new versus control). A genuine effect may be completely obscured or at least be underestimated.

5B. How do we answer the question?
Results section carries the description of number of patients who crossed over and whether contamination was a problem: If so, what was the extent?

5C. How do we interpret the answer?
Ask yourself whether and by how much there will be underestimation of effects due to contamination. Accordingly, exercise caution is interpreting the results.

Q.6. Was the Compliance Adequate?

Compliance refers to the extent to which the study participants adhere to the prescribed interventions.

6A. Why do we ask this question?
Compliance is important because in placebo-controlled studies if the study participants do not take the prescribed intervention, the effects of the intervention would not be seen. If nobody takes the intervention, there would obviously be no effect. The extent to which there will be non-compliance would determine the degree of underestimation of the effects of the intervention. When both arms of the study have active interventions, the difference between the two may be overestimated or underestimated depending on the difference in compliance to the two interventions (details of this aspect is beyond the scope of this book). The papers should also describe the reasons for non-compliance given by the patients – for example, due to intolerable side effects or lack of any perceived benefit. This itself may be an important outcome for some interventions. Tolerability (or acceptability) may be an important criterion for making choices between various interventions of similar efficacy.

6B. How do we answer the question?
The papers should describe the methods of measuring and the extent of compliance in the relevant sections of the paper. Sometimes, the interventions consist of only one injection (e.g. streptokinase in myocardial infarction) or few injections during hospital stay (e.g. dexamethasone for acute bacterial meningitis). In such situations, papers may not describe compliance in any detail.

6C. How do we interpret the answer?
In placebo-controlled studies, if the intervention turns out to be superior to placebo, then compliance is not a major issue, though there would be underestimation of both beneficial and adverse effects of the intervention. If intervention turns out to be ineffective, then one possible reason could be non-compliance. In both cases, tolerability and safety aspects are important and hence reasons for non-compliance should be noted.

Q.7. Was the Follow-Up Complete or Adequate?

Follow-up is said to be complete if the primary outcome(s) for all the patients who entered the study is known. Patients whose status with respect to the primary outcome is unknown are treated as 'lost to follow-up'.

7A. Why do we ask this question?
We ask this question because if losses to follow-up are beyond certain level, the validity of results may be severely compromised and conclusions may be misleading. The reason is that those lost to follow-up tend to have different outcomes than those who are retained.

7B. How do we answer the question?
Usually a table in the study gives the number of patients followed up along with their outcomes. If all patients who entered the study were also followed up, there is no problem. Even if one or few patients are lost to follow-up in studies with

hundreds of patients, there is no problem. The problem comes if the patients lost to follow-up are too many to allow valid conclusions.

7C. How do we interpret the answer?
This requires answering the question – how many are too many? Well, it depends on the total sample size of the study as well as the degree of observed difference in outcomes between the two study groups. Certainly, less than five out of hundreds and less than tens in thousands are unlikely to be too many in any circumstance. But, best thing is to ask: Do the losses to follow-up threaten the validity of the results? Reanalysing the results with certain assumptions for those lost to follow-up can assess this. Such reanalyses are called sensitivity analyses. The type of assumption depends on the study conclusions. If the conclusion favours the new treatment, assume a worse-case scenario and reanalyse. If the conclusion does not favour the new treatment, assume a best-case scenario and reanalyse. (If the comparison is between two active treatments, do both.) The details are as follows:

(i) *Worst-case analysis:* Consider a hypothetical randomised study, which has 100 patients in each of the treatment and control groups, of whom 10 (10 %) are lost to follow-up in each group. Of the remaining 90 patients in each group, 40 (44 %) die in control group and 20 (22 %) in experimental treatment group. The difference (40/90 vs. 20/90) between the two is statistically significant ($P=0.001$). The conclusion is that treatment works. The worst-case scenario analysis will count 40 (40 %) deaths in the control group (all the 10 patients lost to follow-up are assumed to have survived in this group) and 30 (30 %) deaths in the treatment group (all the 10 patients lost to follow-up in this group died). The reanalysis (40/100 vs. 30/100) shows the difference is statistically nonsignificant ($P=0.18$). The conclusion now would be that the difference might be due to chance. Since the two conclusions (one without counting the losses to follow-up and second with worst-case scenario) differ, the losses to follow-up (10 % in this example) are too many to allow strong conclusions. (There is no need to do best-case scenario here because this will lead to the same conclusion as the analysis presented in the study.)
Obviously this analysis is based on an extreme assumption, which is unlikely to be true. In other words, this is a stringent test. If the study passes this test, there is no question that conclusions are valid in spite of losses to follow-up. If the study fails this test, it may or may not be valid; we don't know.

(ii) *Best-case analysis:* If a study concludes that the new treatment does not make any difference but had losses to follow-up, you can do best-case scenario analysis to determine if losses were too many to allow valid conclusions.
Again, consider a hypothetical randomised study with 100 patients in each of the two arms. Let's say, 25 patients in the treatment arm and 20 in the placebo arm were lost to follow-up. Thirty died in each group. The result says there is no statistically significant difference between the two groups; in fact percentage wise, control group is marginally better. The best-case scenario would consider that all those lost to follow-up in the treatment group survived, whereas those in the control group died. The final figures would be 30 deaths in the treatment group and 50 in the control group (now out of 100 in each group).

A reanalysis gives a *P* value of 0.006, statistically very significant difference. This will mean that the losses to follow-up are so many that the results reported in the study may not be called robust.

Of course, the worst- and best-case scenarios are unlikely to be true. They have value if they do not change the conclusions of the studies. (This means conclusions are robust and losses to follow-up do not invalidate the results.) If they do, then validity of the results cannot be said to be robust. The extent to which the validity is compromised depends on the degree to which the outcome of treatment patients lost to follow-up differs from that of control patients lost to follow-up.

Q.8. Correct Outcome Measurement (Was Outcome Measured by Blinded Assessors?)

Correct here means unlikely to be biased. Sometimes, this may not require blinded assessors (e.g. measuring death), but most of the time, blinding is necessary to avoid bias.

8A. Why do we ask this question?
This question is important in studies in which assessor's judgment is required to measure the outcome. If the assessors are aware of the group allocation, they may follow up one group or another more closely and report outcome events more frequently. If the outcome is morbidity, quality of life or activities of daily living, the interpretations of patients' answers may be influenced by the knowledge of the group allocation. However, if the outcome is clear like the all-cause mortality or generalised tonic–clonic seizure, then blinding is less crucial.

8B. How do we answer the question?
Methods section of the paper should describe whether outcome assessment was blinded.

8C. How do we interpret the answer?
Consider the nature of outcome. If it is such that decision cannot be influenced by unblinded assessors (e.g. all-cause mortality), then validity is not threatened. If outcome measurements involve judgment, then consider whether unblinded outcome measurement would favour the treatment (overestimation of benefit) or the control (underestimation).

Q.9. Credible Analysis/Was the Analysis Based on Intention-to- Treat Principle?

9A. Why do we ask this question?
In the basic concepts, you have already read why do we ask this question (Chap. 3).

9B. How do we answer the question?
You may read the methods section to check whether authors indicate that they would use intention-to-treat analysis. If they do so, you may think they did so. Unfortunately, this is not true. Authors carry different notions about ITT analysis. Many so-called ITT analyses are pseudo-ITT. A true ITT analyses would include all patients randomised in the analysis and in their respective groups. This will be apparent in some tables, which contain the primary outcome data and their analysis. Most studies present a study profile, also called trial profile, which indicates how many patients were randomised and also analysed. If you find discrepancy between the number randomised and the number analysed, then read carefully the results section to determine the causes of withdrawals.

9C. How do we interpret the answer?
If the study does not report ITT analysis, look for the reasons. If the withdrawals are due to ineligibility and the withdrawals are unlikely to be biased (e.g. influenced by the knowledge of outcome), you can accept the results. If the withdrawals are due to non-compliance or losses to follow-up, you can do the analysis on ITT basis or do sensitivity analysis and check whether the results change. If they do not, the results are acceptable. If they do, there is a threat to validity.

Summarise the 'validity' assessment by listing the strengths and weakness of the study. Strengths are those validity criteria, which are met. Weaknesses are those criteria, which are not met or unclear. Make a rough judgment of the magnitude of this sum of threats and then decide where does the study fall between hopeless and perfect. If it's hopeless or close to it, there is no point in reading it further. If not, go on to look at the information contained in it.

Q.10. What Are the Results (What Is the Study Saying)?

A number of measures are used to summarise the information: risk difference, risk ratio, etc. (see Chap. 6).

We ask three questions:

(i) Did the new treatment make any difference in the study (See risk ratio, NNT risk difference or odds ratio)? (see Chap. 6)
(ii) If yes, is it likely to be real?
(iii) What is the study's margin of error?

10A. Did the new treatment make any difference?
Look at the type of outcome. Does it have only two possible categories (dichotomous), that means yes/no and death/survival type of outcome, or it is a numerical (termed 'continuous')?

For dichotomous outcomes, look at the % with (or without) the outcome in the treatment and control groups. Usually, the unfavourable outcome is counted. Find out the difference between the control and treatment group (control minus treatment). If it is in 'minus', then treatment seems to be better than control, but if the difference (control minus treatment) is in 'plus', then the treatment seems worse than control (For more details, see Chap. 5).

10B. Is the observed difference real or by chance?
Here we look at the P value (for details see Chap. 3).

10C. What is the study's margin of error?
For this we look at the confidence interval (for details see Chap. 3).

Applicability and Application

Are the study results applicable in (our) practice?

This requires examining the relevance of population, intervention, comparison and outcomes (PICO) in the study to your practice or your patient:

1. *Is the study population relevant to my practice or patients?*
   Here you need to examine the eligibility (inclusion and exclusion) criteria of the study subjects and sometimes also their baseline characteristics. Some degree of judgment has to be exercised. If your patient is one year older or younger than the age limits of the eligibility criteria, it may not be right to say that the study population is irrelevant to my patient. To conclude irrelevance, there should be a compelling reason, usually one which makes the prognosis very different in your patient or which contraindicates the use of intervention or makes it futile. This judgment calls on your background knowledge of the field.
2. *Is the intervention relevant?*
   Relevant here means available, affordable, acceptable and feasible. If the intervention is not available, the whole exercise is only of academic value. The intervention should also be affordable, acceptable and feasible. Some interventions are culturally not acceptable. For example, liver or fish oil may be nutritious, but in some strictly vegetarian communities, this may not be acceptable. Sometimes an intervention is not feasible. For example, there may not be a well-equipped operation theatre even if a vascular surgeon is available to do carotid endarterectomy.
3. *Is the comparison relevant?*
   Sometimes, studies are conducted with unacceptable treatment in the background or as control. In both situations, the results are of doubtful applicability to situations when the standard treatment is different. For example, Lebel et al [1] studied the effectiveness of dexamethasone with cefuroxime as the background treatment in children with acute bacterial meningitis (ABM). Cefuroxime has been shown to be inferior to ceftriaxone or cefotaxime in ABM and is not recommended for use in the condition. Even though dexamethasone was found to reduce the risk of deafness, one did not know whether the same results would apply when ceftriaxone or cefotaxime was used as the background treatment (later the benefit was shown also in presence of ceftriaxone or cefotaxime). Similarly, let us say a new drug is shown to be effective in a condition. Thereafter,

several compounds, some very expensive, of the same class of drugs become available usually from different companies; the relevant question is whether the more expensive ones are better than the less expensive ones, and accordingly, we need to look for studies involving such comparisons, not only the ones comparing each of the new compounds against placebos. For example, there are many studies comparing ACE inhibitors in preventing progression of diabetic nephropathy; each one is more effective than placebo. But range of their cost is so wide that the relevant question is whether the more expensive ones are better than inexpensive ones. Unfortunately such comparative studies are few or non-existent.

4. *Are all the clinically relevant (meaningful) outcomes measured?*
This is probably the most crucial element in judging relevance. You should ask: What are the investigators trying to achieve? Will the achievements persuade me and my patients to adopt the intervention? Will they be meaningful from the patients' point of view? Certain outcomes are clearly meaningful to all concerned, for example, decreased mortality or improvement in quality of life and independence in activities of daily living, but some outcomes are only intermediate outcomes, e.g. CSF normalisation in meningitis or suppressed arrhythmia in acute myocardial infarction. Encainide successfully suppressed arrhythmias but increased mortality [2, 3]. In general, intermediate outcomes are rarely clinically relevant as well as meaningful (see also Chap. 9).
The second types of outcomes, which require exercising caution, are scale-based outcomes. Often, investigators compare the mean (or median) scores of the experimental and control groups. While there may be statistically significant differences in the mean (or median), one should not assume that they are also clinically meaningful. The magnitude of difference should be examined for its meaning in clinical terms. In many (or most) scales, this clinically meaningful difference is not known. In such instances, treatment success may be defined as achievement of certain scores or as increase (or decrease depending on the scale) by certain levels of scores, and the proportion of patients achieving treatment success may be compared. This will be clearly meaningful from a clinical point of view. Sometimes a certain level of the score defines independence in activities of daily living, and proportions of patients achieving the level are compared to determine both statistical and clinical significance. This is clearly a meaningful approach.

Application

If the study is valid and applicable, results show significant (important) benefit, you decide to apply the new treatment to your patient. First, you estimate (from your clinical experience and knowledge) the baseline risk of unfavourable outcome in your patient. Then determine what would be the risk if the new treatment is given to the patient. Then consider in consultation with the patient whether the benefit is worth the costs, harm and inconvenience. For example, let us consider two patients with intracerebral haemorrhage: one fully conscious and alert with small haematoma and another semi-comatose with large haematoma. You estimate that the risk of unfavourable (bad) outcome (death or disability) is 2 % in the conscious patient and 80 % in the semi-comatose patient. Let us say you are considering surgery as an option and surgery reduces the risk of bad outcome by 10 % (RRR = 10 %). The conscious patient's risk with surgery may decrease from 2 to 1.8 % [10 % of 2 is 0.2 and 2 − 0.2 = 1.8]. Given the risk and cost of surgery, you and your patient decide that surgery is not a worthwhile option. On the other hand, surgery would decrease the risk of bad outcome in the semi-comatose patient from 80 to 72 % (10 % of 80 is 8 and 80 − 8 = 72). In this case, you may discuss with the patient's relatives and decide that surgery is worthwhile. Thus, you can see that even after the overall conclusion (after validity, results and applicability assessment) is in favour of an intervention, you may not prescribe (apply) it to some patients and prescribe to some. Application is one step further after applicability assessment.

References

1. Lebel MH, Freji BJ, Syrogiannopoulos GA, Chrane DF, Hoyt MJ, Stewart SM, et al. Dexamethasone therapy for bacterial meningitis: results of two double-blind, placebo-controlled trials. N Engl J Med. 1988;319:964–71.
2. Echt DS, Liebson PR, Mitchell LB, et al. Mortality and morbidity in patients receiving encainide, flecainide, or placebo: the Cardiac Arrhythmia Suppression Trial. N Engl J Med. 1991;324:781–8.
3. The Cardiac Arrhythmia Suppression Trial II Investigators. Effect of the antiarrhythmic agent moricizine on survival after myocardial infarction. N Engl J Med. 1992;327:227–33.

Further Reading

Byington RP, Curb JD, Mattson ME. Assessment of double-blindness at the conclusion of the beta-Blocker Heart Attack Trial. JAMA. 1985;253:1733–6.

Guyatt G, Rennie D, editors. User's guides to the medical literature: a manual for evidence-based clinical practice. Chicago: AMA Press; 2002. (www.ama-assn.org).

Guyatt GH, Sackett DL, Cook DJ. Users' guides to the medical literature. II. How to use an article about therapy or prevention. A. Are the results of the study valid? Evidence-Based Medicine Working Group. JAMA. 1993;270:2598–601.

Oxman AD, Guyatt GH. A consumer's guide to subgroup analyses. Ann Intern Med. 1992;116:78–84.

Peto R, et al. Design and analysis of randomized clinical trials requiring prolonged observation of each patient. II. Analysis and examples. Br J Cancer. 1977;35:1–39.

Sackett DL, Gent M. Controversy in counting and attributing events in clinical trials. N Engl J Med. 1979;301:1410–2.

Sacks H, Chalmers TC, Smith Jr H. Randomized versus historical controls for clinical trials. Am J Med. 1982;72:233–40.

Schulz KF, Chalmers I, Hayes RJ, Altman DG. Empirical evidence of bias, dimensions of methodological quality associated with estimates of treatment effects in controlled trials. JAMA. 1995;273:408–12.

Yusuf S, Collins R, Peto R. Why do we need some large, simple randomized trials? Stat Med. 1984;3:409–22.

[illegible]

1. [illegible]

[illegible]

[illegible] Reading

[illegible]

Chapter 6
Therapy: Critical Appraisal Part 2 (Interpreting Results)

This chapter deals with the second part of the critical appraisal. We want to know: 'How good is the treatment?' We would love to have one sentence with one figure to answer this question, but in life, one figure is not enough to tell the whole story about many things. For example, we ask our children: How good are your marks? If he says 99 %, we feel happy. But then soon we want to know, is it the best in the class – in other words, what is his/her position relative to the other students. How many students have marks below this? How many have marks above this? This is to know his relative position. This is described in terms of percentile. The per cent of marks in absolute terms is 99, but it is possible that most students had it (the exam was very easy). Some testing services use per cent, percentile, grade (A1, A2, B1, etc.) and GPA (grade point average) to describe the results. Each figure may give a different perspective and may appeal to different constituencies. This is why stock markets always use at least two figures to describe what happened on the day: usually one to describe the difference in actual figures (absolute difference) and one to describe it in per cent terms (relative to the opening figure).

Similarly, to describe the results of a treatment study, we have relative as well absolute measures like risk difference (an absolute measure), risk ratio (relative risk), odds ratio and rate ratio; each one gives a different perspective and appeals to different constituencies. Let us take another example.

Let us consider an announcement by the government: '5,000 doctors working in government hospitals will receive an average increase in salary of 1,000 dollar per month costing 60 million (5 million × 12) dollars per year'. You as a doctor will be happy to hear the news and start calculating how many dollars more you will get per month. The announcement talks about average that does not mean every doctor will get 1,000 dollars more per month. Some doctors may have a current salary of 1,000 dollars per month, while others may have 14,000 dollars per month. To know how much increase you will get, you need another figure that is 'per cent' increase. You ask a government officer: How much is the increase in 'per cent' terms? He tells you that it is 10 % across all doctors. Now you know how much increase you will get per month. Your current 5,000 dollars per month will increase by 500 dollars (10 % of 5,000). So you will get 5,500 dollars per month. This example shows that we need

K. Prasad, *Fundamentals of Evidence-Based Medicine*,
DOI 10.1007/978-81-322-0831-0_6, © Springer India 2013

two kinds of measures for measuring a change: One like average 1,000 dollars increase (or sometimes a decrease in, say, failure rate of a treatment) is a 'difference' measure; and second like 10 % increase is derived from a 'ratio' measure. The difference measure helps to assess impact overall (say, for groups of patients, or in population), while 'ratio' measure helps to asses impact on an individual. (In epidemiology, a difference measure like attributable risk indicates the impact of a risk factor on population, whereas the ratio measure like risk ratio indicates strength of causal relationship.)

Measures of Effect of Treatment

What are the measures? Consider this statement in a newspaper: 'Economic reforms have led to decline in unemployment rate from 20 to 15 %, thus reducing it by 25 %'. You may wonder how a difference of 5 % (20 % – 15 %) translates to a reduction of 25 %. One workshop participant explained it as follows: 'If 20 % is taken as 100, 15 % would be 75 and 5 % would be equal to 25 %'. In medical world, we often use the term 'risk' of mortality, recurrence, etc. Full statement may be, for example, the mortality decreased from 20 % in control group to 15 % in new treatment group, thus showing that the new treatment reduced mortality by 25 %. The terms used are as follows:

20%–15% = 5% Risk difference (RD)
Baseline risk or Control group risk (CGR) 20% = if taken as 100%
then Treatment/experimental group risk (EGR) 15% = 75% or 0.75,
which is also called 'Risk Ratio' or 'Relative Risk (RR)'
Then 5% = 25%, called 'Relative risk reduction (RRR)'

Difference measure is RD (also called 'absolute risk reduction'), which is simply a difference between the two risks (conventionally, EGR – CGR). In this case, (15 % – 20 %) = –5 %. Minus indicates that the risk decreases with the new treatment. If EGR was greater than CGR, the difference will be positive (plus), indicating that the new treatment, in fact, increases the risk. If the risk was the same in both groups, the difference will be '0'. (Please note that all authors do not follow the convention, and hence, the plus or minus sign may not always mean the same in all papers. Always look at the risk in individual groups to decide what the new treatment does.)

'Ratio' measure is RR = 75 % (usually expressed in decimals as 0.75). So, how do you get risk ratio? Simply by taking a ratio of experimental group risk to control group risk (EGR/CGR). This will give you RR in decimals (multiply by 100 to get per cent).

From RR, you can easily find out 'per cent' change RRR = 25 % (100 – 75 or 1 – 0.75). In other words, 1 – RR (in decimals) or (100 – RR) in % gives you RRR.

The formula may be written as

In decimals, RRR = 1 – RR
In percent, RRR (%) 100 – RR (%)

If only 'difference' and 'baseline risk' or CGR is given, you can find out RRR by dividing the difference with baseline risk and multiplying it by 100. The formula may be written as

$$\text{Relative risk reduction (RRR) in\%} = \frac{\text{Risk difference (RD)}}{\text{Baseline risk or control group risk}} \times 100$$

NNT (Number Needed to Treat)

You can find out NNT from risk difference. Risk difference of −5 % means 5 less (minus) deaths per 100 patients treated. In other words, for avoiding five deaths we need to treat 100 patients. Therefore, for one death to be avoided, the number needed to treat is 100/5 = 20. We can easily see the relationship. 5 % in fraction terms is 5/100, whereas number need to treat (NNT) is 100/5. So, what we can do to find out NNT? Three steps: First, find out the difference in risk; second, write this in the form of a fraction (obviously with denominator as 100); and third, invert the fraction so that you have 100 in the numerator and the difference (in %) in the denominator. Do the cancellation and rounding. The figure you get is the number needed to treat. If you like decimals you can do in two steps: First find out the risk difference or ARR (say, 0.05). Then take its inverse, that is, 1/risk difference or 1/ARR.

Whenever you talk of NNT, you must specify the follow-up period over which the difference was observed and the unfavourable outcome, which was avoided. NNT usually makes sense only when the treatment has been shown to make a statistically significant difference.

How much NNT is good? Well, there is no magic figure. For an inexpensive drug with no side effect, acceptable NNT may be 100 or even 200, whereas for risky surgery it may be only 20. Acceptable NNTs may be different for prophylactic versus 'active treatments'. As a general guide, for active treatments, the acceptable NNT may be 20 or 25, whereas for preventive treatments, even 250 or 500. To give you some idea about NNTs, I present a table of NNTs for commonly used treatment (Table 6.1).

Interpretation of Measures of Effect of Treatment

If the new treatment has no effect, the risk (of mortality) in both groups will be the same, say, 20 %. The difference will be '0' (20 % − 20 %), and the ratio will be '1' (20 %/20 %). If the new treatment decreases the risk, the difference will be negative, and if it increases, it will be positive. The ratio (RR), if the treatment is effective, will be less than 1 (in our example, 15 %/20 % = 0.75), and if new treatment increases the risk (say, to 25 %), it will be more than 1 (25 %/20 % = 1.25). All ratio measures

Table 6.1 NNTs for commonly used interventions in medicine

Condition	Treatment	Duration of treatment	Comparator	Outcome	NNT
Angina	Isosorbide dinitrate	4–6 weeks	Placebo	Prevention exercise-induced angina	5.0
Anticipated preterm delivery	Corticosteroids	Before delivery	No treatment	Risk of foetal RDS	11
Asthma (childhood)	Budesonide and formoterol	1 year	Budesonide alone	Free of severe exacerbation for 1 year	11
Diabetic neuropathy	Anticonvulsants			50 % pain relief	2.5
Dementia	Gingko	1 year	Placebo	ADAS-Cog 4 points better	7.9
Head lice	Permethrin	14 days	Placebo	Cure	1.1
Hypertension in the elderly	Drug treatments	At least 1 year	No treatment	Overall prevention of cardiovascular event over 5 years	18
Primary prevention	Various	5 years	No treatment	Prevent one myocardial infarction or cerebrovascular death	69
Secondary prevention	Various	5 years	No treatment	Prevent one myocardial infarction or cerebrovascular death	16
Migraine	Subcutaneous sumatriptan	Single dose	Placebo	Headache relieved at 2 h	2.0
Migraine	Oral sumatriptan	Single dose	Placebo	Headache relieved at 2 h	2.6
Myocardial infarction	Aspirin plus streptokinase	1 H I.V. infusion of streptokinase, 1 month of oral aspirin	No treatment	Five-week vascular mortality, prevent one death	20
Peptic ulcer	Triple therapy	6–10 weeks	Histamine antagonist	*H. pylori* eradication	1.1
Peptic ulcer	Triple therapy	6–10 weeks	Histamine antagonist	Ulcers remaining cured at 1 year	1.8
Prostate – benign hypertrophy	Finasteride	2 years	Placebo	Prevent one operation	39
MRC 17,354 individuals 36–64 years diastolic 90–109 mmHg	Benzofluazide propranolol	5.5 years	Placebo	Prevent one stroke at 1 year	850
CATS 1,072 patients 1 week to 4 months after stroke	Ticlopidine	2 years	Placebo		15
ESPS2 6,602 patients >18 years TIA or stroke in previous 3 months	Aspirin	2 years	Placebo		37
	Dipyridamole				42
	Aspirin plus Dipyridamole				8

behave in the same way. (Please note that even with effective treatment, one could take the ratio as 20 %/15 % = 1.33 (more than 1), but most authors follow the above convention and show ratio measure less than 1, when the new treatment decreases the risk. Again, not all authors follow the convention, and you need to carefully look at the figures.)

Please remember, all the time we are thinking that the treatment decreases the risk. Sometimes, treatments are harmful. They increase the risk. In this case, what we will get is the number needed to treat to cause one extra death or harm. So, you must see what the treatment is doing. Accordingly, interpret the NNT. But you know that even effective and helpful treatments have downsides as well. We can find out NNT to prevent one adverse outcome or NNT to cause one extra harm (side effect or adverse effect). The latter is sometimes called *NNH (Number needed to harm)*.

To recapitulate, we have covered four measures of treatment effect in our example: (1) risk difference (RD) or Absolute Risk Reduction (ARR) = −5 %, or −0.05; (2) NNT = 20; (3) RR (risk ratio or relative risk) = 80 % or 0.0; and (4) relative risk reduction (RRR) = 20 % or 0.2.

The measures *RD (ARR), NNT, RR and RRR* are generally adequate for communication among clinicians and are enough to deal with most situations. But sometimes, like in case–control studies, none of the measures apply. The measure, which applies to this kind of studies as well as all others, is based on odds (unlike all of the above which are based on probabilities or risks).

Odds Ratio

We often say odds of England team winning the cricket match is 1:4. What does it mean? It means: If there is one chance of winning, there are four chances of losing – in other words, one in five (20 %) chance of winning and four in five (80 %) chance of losing. Chance is probability. Odds of 1:4 means 20 % probability of winning and 80 % probability of losing. Thus, odds looks at both sides of the coin – win versus lose, death versus survival and improvement versus deterioration. Odds of 1:4 is equal to ¼, that is, 0.25 or 25 %. You can see that 25 % odds of winning means 20 % probability of winning. You need not bother about this interrelationship. All you need to remember is that odds expression requires probability of one side of the coin (e.g. winning) in the numerator and probability of the other side of coin (losing, in our example) in the denominator.

Consider an example. Let us say 20 % of the patients in the treatment group died, which means 80 % survived in the treatment group. So, what is odds of death in the treatment group. Remember, for odds we will have to have chance (probability) of death in the numerator, that is, 20 %, and chance of survival in the denominator, that is, 80 %. So, odds will be 20 %/80 % (in decimals, 0.2/0.8). This is equal to 1/4.

Now, let us say 25 % of the patients in the control group died, which means 75 % survived. So, odds of death in the control group is 25 %/75 % (or 0.25/0.75) = 1/3.

Therefore, *odds ratio* which usually has odds of death (or any adverse event) in the treatment group as the numerator and odds of death in the placebo group in the denominator will be equal to $1/4/1/3 = 1/4 \div 1/3 = 1/4 \times 3/1 = 3/4 = 0.75$ (or 75 %). Thus, one of expressing the treatment effect is odds ratio = 0.75 (=75 %). Again OR can be interpreted as 'odds remaining'. So odds remaining is 75 %. Therefore, odds reduction is (100–75) % = 25 %.

Summary

Treatment effect in our example can be expressed in several ways:

(a) Risk of death is decreased from 25 to 20 %.
(b) *Risk difference* or *absolute risk reduction* is −5 % (5/100).
(c) *NNT* is 100/5, i.e. 20.
(d) *Risk ratio or relative risk* = 20 %/25 % = 0.8 or 80 %.
(e) *Relative risk reduction* = 20 %.
(f) *Odds ratio* = 0.75 or 75 %.
(g) *Odds reduction* is 25 %.

If you are the drug manufacturer, what will be your choicest measure? Obviously odds reduction of 25 %. What will be your second choice? Relative risk reduction of 20 %. Both are relative to the odds or risks in the control group (which is taken as 100 %), which will be reduced by 25 or 20 %, respectively. In actual terms, how much difference does the treatment make? Only 5 %. This is well captured by NNT, i.e. 20 persons need to be treated to prevent one extra death. All are technically correct measures each giving one perspective on the effect of the treatment.

Why There Are So Many Effect Measures (Relative Merits and Demerits)?

Different people may look at the same result for different purposes and in different ways. I am sure you have seen this many times in patient's investigation results. Consider a brain CT of a patient suspected to have hemorrhagic stroke. Emergency physician looks at the CT to see if this confirms his suspicion. If yes, he refers the case to a neurologist. The neurologist looks at it to determine whether the site is typical of a hypertensive bleed and calculates the volume of the haematoma to inform the patient or relatives about his prognosis. If he thinks that the prognosis with medical treatment alone is not favourable, then he refers the case to a neurosurgeon who tries to determine whether the haematoma is operable or what is the benefit versus risk of surgery in this haematoma (there are many other issues, but let us use only the above for illustration). Similarly, the results of a study have many clients. Each client has a different purpose in mind when he looks at the results.

Let us consider a study that compared the treatment of stroke in 'stroke unit' versus 'general medical ward'. The results have many clients with different objectives in mind.

1. Hospital administration wants to know the cost-effectiveness of stroke unit as compared with the current treatment policy of treating stroke patients in general medical ward.
2. The physician wants to know how much benefit it would offer to his patients. He sees different kinds of patients. Some patients are young with few risk factors and mild stroke, say, with 2 % risk of institutionalisation. Some patients are old with many risk factors and severe stroke with (say) 90 % risk of death or dependence. The physician wants to know the benefit in each type of patients.

Accordingly, we want effect measures which:

1. Are easy to understand
2. Give some idea about cost-effectiveness
3. Are meaningfully applicable for all kinds of patients
4. Convey the same idea whether you measure unfavourable (e.g. death) or favourable (e.g. survival) outcome

Number Need to Treat (NNT)

Let us say the results of a study showed that 50 % of stroke patients treated in the general medical ward (hereinafter called 'ward') were institutionalised, whereas only 25 % were so in the group treated in a stroke unit (assume both had similar mortality). Thus, stroke unit made a difference of – 25 % (25 % – 50 %), yielding an NNT of 4. This means 4 patients need to be treated in stroke unit to avoid one institutionalisation in patients with stroke.

The hospital administrator calculates how much the stroke unit would cost. If on an average it is $5,000, he can easily see that $20,000 needs to be spent to prevent one institutionalisation. He can easily compare the cost of institutionalisation versus stroke unit treatment and take a decision. Thus, one advantage of NNT is that it gives a quick (even if dirty) idea about cost-effectiveness.

It has another advantage. This becomes apparent when we are dealing with a very low frequency of outcome. For example, mammography programmes for 7 years reduce the incidence of death from breast cancer from 0.08 to 0.02 %, a difference of 0.06 %. NNT turns out to be 1,666. This means 1,666 ladies need to have regular mammography for 7 years to prevent one death from breast cancer. You may find saying this easier and more understandable than a difference of 0.06 %. Thus, NNT helps to convert a small decimal into a round figure, which can be easily understood and also pronounced (saves your tongue). Thus, two advantages of NNT are:

(i) Provides easy way to get an idea of cost-benefit
(ii) More easily understood by policymakers and physician

But NNT has disadvantages too:

(i) For example, if you are communicating with the patient and, say, four patients need to be treated to save one additional patient, the patient might ask: Am I likely to be one of the saved or among the three dead? In other words, this is not easily interpretable by an individual patient.

Risk Difference (RD) or ARR (Absolute Risk Reduction)

Risk difference has three merits:

(i) Easy to calculate and interpret: You have to do only a subtraction; RD tells you how much difference the intervention could make.
(ii) It is symmetrical, i.e. conveys the same effect whether you measure the favourable or unfavourable outcome. In the stroke example, if you measured the favourable outcome like 'going home', still the difference will be the same. 50 % went home in the 'ward' group and 75 % in the stroke unit group – a difference of 25 %, which is the same in magnitude as earlier.
(iii) It helps in the calculation of NNT.
(iv) The fourth merit of RD is that its confidence interval can be calculated even when no patient had the outcome of interest in any group. For example, no patient died in any group (no need to elaborate in this book).

However, it has some demerits:

(i) Sometimes, it is too small to be pronounced and interpreted easily (e.g. see mammography example above).
(ii) It cannot apply equally to all types of patients. Consider the two patients with acute stroke – one mild and one severe. You might think (though it is not correct) that the severe patient's risk of death/institutionalisation would be down to 65 % (90–25), but what about the mild patient – as such his risk is 2 %. How can stroke unit make a difference of 25 %, when the total risk is 2 %. This illustrates the difficulty in using the RD (or ARR) from the study data (however, RR is equally applicable in both cases – see below).

Risk Ratio or Relative Risk (RR)

It has the merit of applicability to all kinds of patients. For example, in the stroke example RR would be 25 %/50 % = 0.5 (=50 %). That means risk with treatment in stroke unit is 50 % of that with treatment in general medical ward. Thus, it would be 45 % (half of 90) with the stroke unit treatment in the severe case, whereas it would be 1 % (half of two per cent) in the mild case. RR easily applies to both.

However, the demerit in RR is that it's not symmetrical. Above you have seen the stroke unit halves the risk of unfavourable. If you measure favourable outcome here (like 'going home'), then it should double its rate, but no. With 75 % going home in the stroke unit group and 50 % in the ward treatment group, RR of 'going home' is 75 %/50 % = 1.5, rather than two. The other demerit which you might have noticed is that it does not sound right to say risk of 'going home'. Going home is a favourable outcome, and risk is a rather loaded concept which sounds awkward in association with favourable outcome.

To summarise, merits of RR is:

(i) Applicability to all kinds of patients
(ii) Easier to interpret than odds ratio

Its demerits are:

(i) Asymmetry: if there is 10 % risk of death in experimental group and 40 % in control group, RR = 0.25, i.e. RRR = 1 − 0.25 = 0.75, or 75 % risk reduction. If we counted survival, risk of survival in experimental group will be 90 % and in control group 60 %; RR = 1.5, that means relative risk increase of survival is 50 %. You can see that one way it is 75 %, the other way 50 %. This is the asymmetry.
(ii) Lack of neutrality: Risk of survival sounds awkward. Risk sounds alright only for unfavourable outcomes, not favourable ones. So this is not a neutral concept.
(iii) There is no way to calculate confidence interval of RR when there is zero event in both the treatment groups, for example, no death in any of the two groups in a study.

Odds Ratio

The merits of OR is that:

(i) Like RR, it is applicable to all kinds of patients, irrespective of their level of risk without the treatment.
(ii) It is not a loaded concept. It's neutral. Odds of going home sounds as appropriate as odds of institutionalisation or death. Just as odds of winning or losing both sound acceptable.
(iii) It is symmetrical. In the stroke example, the odds of institutionalisation in the 'stroke unit' group is 50:50 = 1, whereas in the 'general ward' group, it is 75:25 = 3. The odds ratio for institutionalisation with stroke unit versus general ward is 1/3. Now, let us see what happens if we measured odds of going home. This is 50:50 (=1) with stroke unit group and 25:75 with the general ward group, or 1/3. Therefore, odds ratio of going home is $1 \div (1/3) = 1 \times (3/1) = 3$. Thus, odds of institutionalisation with stroke unit care is 1/3 of that with general ward. Similarly odds of going home with stroke unit is three times that

with general ward. The symmetry is clear and no matter what you measure – the favourable or unfavourable outcome – it gives the same impression.

(iv) The fourth merit of OR is that it can be used in one of the commonest forms of adjusted analysis (using logistic regression), whereas RD or RR cannot be.

(v) It has certain mathematical properties that make it a favoured measure for some statistical calculations including meta-analysis.

The demerits of OR are that:

(i) It is a difficult concept to understand and interpret for health professionals.

(ii) If interpreted like RR, it overestimates the treatment effects. OR and RR are similar only when events in the control and experimental group are 10 % or less or when they are close to one.

(iii) Like that in RR, there is no way to calculate the confidence interval around OR, when there is zero event in both the treatment arms. Only RD lends itself to calculation of C.I. in this situation.

Which One Should a Clinician Use?

It is generally enough to know that the RD, NNT, RR and RRR are associated with a treatment. OR may be treated as RR when events in the experimental and control group are 10 % or less. Otherwise, there are formulae (available on the Internet) to convert OR in RR or NNT.

Further Reading

Guyatt G, Rennie D, editors. User's guides to the medical literature: a manual for evidence-based clinical practice. Chicago: AMA Press; 2002. (www.ama-assn.org).

Laupacis A, Sackett DL, Roberts RS. An assessment of clinically useful measures of the consequences of treatment. N Engl J Med. 1988;318:1728–33.

Malenka DJ, Baron JA, Johansen S, Wahrenberger JW, Ross JM. The framing effect of relative and absolute risk. J Gen Intern Med. 1993;8:543–8.

Naylor CD, Chen E, Strauss B. Measured enthusiasm : does the method of reporting trial results alter perceptions of therapeutic effectiveness? Ann Intern Med. 1992;117:916–21.

Peto R, et al. Design and analysis of randomized clinical trials requiring prolonged observation of each patient. II. Analysis and examples. Br J Cancer. 1977;35:1–39.

Chapter 7
Diagnostic Test: Fundamental Concepts

The Clinical Diagnostic Process

Clinical diagnosis is sometimes a spot diagnosis, but more often a matter of pattern recognition and probabilistic thinking. Usually, making a diagnosis is moving from possibilities to high or low probabilities. Based on history and physical examination, we think of one or more possibilities. Some, we think, are more likely than others, while some may have to be ruled out. We do diagnostic tests to increase the probability of more likely ones to nearly 95 % or above and decrease the probability of the 'rule out' diagnoses to near 'zero' or less than 5 %. Thus, the function of a diagnostic test is to increase or decrease (in one word, *revise*) the probability of the diseases under consideration. The probability of a disease we consider before ordering a diagnostic test (called 'pretest probability') should substantially change after the test. The probability we get after the test result is called 'posttest probability'. Pretest probability is usually based on history and physical examination. In fact, it develops through several revisions, starting with some probability with the first symptom and changing the probability as newer findings emerge on history and physical examination. For example, as soon as a patient complains of chest pain of 2 h of duration (without history of trauma), we think of certain possibilities – like acute myocardial infarction (MI), pericarditis, pneumonia, pleurisy and dissection of aorta. Looking at his age of, say, 60 years, and considering the frequency, we think MI more likely than others. We ask about the characteristics of pain (onset, character, radiation, etc.) and risk factors (like diabetes, hypertension, smoking, hyperlipidemia) and accordingly revise the probability of MI to a high level (say, 60 %). Then we do certain tests like ECG and serum CPK or Trop-T. Each revises the probability further. If CK and ECG changes are borderline, the probability may not change much, but if ECG shows ST–T changes, the probability goes up, and if CK is also raised 2× normal, then the probability is nearly 99–100 % and the diagnosis is confirmed. The tests in this case are revising the pretest probability of 60 % to a posttest probability of 99–100 %. The example illustrates that the function of a diagnostic test is to revise the pretest probability of the diseases which are being considered in the differential diagnosis (Table 7.1).

K. Prasad, *Fundamentals of Evidence-Based Medicine*,
DOI 10.1007/978-81-322-0831-0_7, © Springer India 2013

Table 7.1 Steps in making a diagnosis (probabilistic method)

Steps	Process of diagnosis
1.	Collect initial information (from history or examination)
2.	Generate possibilities
3.	Attach probability to each possibility
4.	Collect more information
5.	Revise probabilities
6.	Perform diagnostic tests
7.	Revise probabilities further to a level that helps decision-making

The function of a diagnostic test is to revise pretest probabilities of the diseases under consideration to posttest probabilities.

Dichotomous and Multilevel Results

What revises the pretest probability? The test results. Test results may take a number of forms: Sometimes they are numbers like erythrocyte sedimentation rate (ESR); sometimes they are multiple categories – strongly positive, moderately positive, mild or borderline positive and negative or strongly negative. Even the results expressed in numbers are most of the time converted in our mind into multiple categories: very high, high, borderline high, normal, borderline low, very low, etc. Both the forms may be termed 'multilevel results'. At other times, results are expressed as positive and negative, termed dichotomous results. No matter how the results are expressed, they are useful only if they revise pretest probability to such a level of posttest probability that helps us to make a decision about the next step, for example, in treatment (i.e. helps to cross the treatment threshold). The usefulness of a test depends on whether its results help in treatment decision-making. A test is only as good as its results. Every type of test result needs to be assessed – whether a strongly positive, moderately positive or negative. Even if one of the results is helpful, the test may be considered useful.

More on Pretest Probabilities, Posttest Probabilities and Predictive Values

Let us start with a scenario. You want to develop a facility to determine foetal sex using ultrasound. You come across two ultrasonographers who claim to be correct nearly always in sex determination of foetus at 14 weeks' gestation. You discuss and decide to conduct a study to establish the facility. You buy a state-of-the-art ultrasound machine, which gives 3-D picture of the foetus. Ultrasound is an operator-dependent technology. First you decide to establish the consistency of the ultrasonographers (US) – both interobserver and intraobserver. Same patients are

Table 7.2 Accuracy of ultrasound prediction of male foetus

	Actual at birth		Posttest probability	
	Male	Female	Male (%)	Female (%)
Test result predicts – male 210	189	21	90	10

tested twice by the same observer (without his knowledge) and some by both the observers independently. Interobserver and intraobserver consistency are examined and you find them acceptable.

The next question is how to check their correctness. It was clear that the US report had to be compared with the final diagnosis at birth. You verify the US findings with diagnosis at birth in 400 consecutive births. Let us look at the results. Well, before you look at the results, think for a moment. Suppose US prediction of male was found correct in 60 % and of females 65 %. Do you think it is good? Surely not. As such without any test, what do you guess is the chance (probability) of male babies, 50 %, and of female babies, 50 %. Therefore, after the test if the chance becomes 60 or 65 %, this cannot be called acceptable, because any decision on the basis of such prediction or even communication to the patient is far too often wrong. You want the probabilities after the test to be much more (say, 90–99 %) than the probabilities before the test (which is 50 %). Probabilities before the test are called 'pretest probabilities' and those after the test results, 'posttest probabilities'. A good test should give good results. Good results are those which revise pretest probabilities to such an extent that correct decisions can be taken or correct information can be given to patients.

In our scenario, there are two pretest probabilities. One for male and one for female, both in this case are 50 %. Let us see what the US can predict based on the test result. His predictions may be male or female. But it can't be 100 % correct. You need to know what per cent of his male predictions are correct and similarly what predictions of his female predictions are correct. Let us take them one by one. Suppose that in 400 pregnancies he predicted 210 to be male, of which 189 turned out to be correct (Table 7.2). Thus, what per cent of his 'male' predictions is correct? 189/210 = 0.9 = 90 %. This means, in the next patient if he predicts male, the probability of male baby is approximately 90 %. This is posttest probability. But what happens to the rest of the 10 %. The US predicted male but they actually turned out to be female. Thus, if test prediction is male, the posttest probability of male is 90 % and that of female is 10 %.

Now let us see what happened to 'female' predictions. Of 190 predicted female, 179 turned out to be correct. Thus, what per cent of female predictions were correct? 179/190 = 0.94 = 94 %. Thus, in the next patient if he predicts female, the probability (posttest) that the baby will be female is approximately 94 %. Again, what about 6 % – this is the posttest probability of male if US predicted female. Therefore, if test prediction is female, the posttest probability of female is 94 % and that of male is 6 % (Table 7.3).

Combining Tables 7.2 and 7.3 and calling the 'at birth' examination as gold standard result gives us a complete table (Table 7.4).

Table 7.3 Accuracy of ultrasound prediction of female foetus

	Actual at birth		Posttest probability	
	Female	Male	Male (%)	Female (%)
Test result predicts – female 190	179	11	6	94

Table 7.4 2x2 table of accuracy ultrasound prediction of foetal sex

			Gold standard result (actual)		Posttest probability	
			Male	Female	Male (%)	Female (%)
Test result	Male	210	189	21	90	10
	Female	190	11	179	6	94

Thus, you can see that there are four posttest probabilities, but the second can be easily derived if we know any one of the posttest probability for male or female. You can also see that they are actually correctness of each test prediction, and the predictions are of value only if they are correct. They are also called 'predictive values'. Since clinical tests are usually reported as positive or negative, there are 'positive predictive values' and 'negative predictive values'. If you take male as 'positive' and female as 'negative', the posttest probability of male with test result positive (predicting male) will be called 'positive predictive value', and the posttest probability of female with test result negative (predicting female) will be called 'negative predictive value'. This is all we need to know about the test in this situation. We have all the necessary information for using the test in our practice, except that we may keep some margin of error in mind with these figures (for further discussion on margin of error, see chapter 4 section on confidence intervals).

You may ask, what about sensitivity and specificity? Well, you don't need them in this situation. All you need to know is the prediction correctness or predictive values of your US. If you know that when US says male, 90 % chance that it will be male, and similarly if he says female, 94 % chance it will be female, then you have all the necessary information for use. What matters while using the information is the predictive values – not sensitivity or specificity. But this is because the example is unique. The pretest probability (sometimes also called 'prevalence') is 50 % male (or 50 % female) in all populations, all hospitals around the world. But, the disease prevalence changes from one place to another, even in one hospital population to another. When this happens, the predictive values change remarkably and you need something, which is relatively stable across populations, and this is where sensitivity and specificity are helpful. Further discussion on this follows in the next section.

Sensitivity and Specificity

Let us start with a story. A chairman of accident and emergency got concerned with what appeared to be overdiagnosis of acute appendicitis. Many patients operated in emergency were found to have normal appendix. Over the last 3 years, year after

Table 7.5 2x2 table of accuracy of ultrasound diagnosis of appendicitis in a hypothetical study

	Total	Disease +ve	Disease –ve
US+	28	25 (89 %)	3 (11 %)
US–	172	15 (9 %)	157 (91 %)

year only 20 % of patients suspected to have appendicitis had actually inflamed appendix on pathological examination. [This 20 % is called 'prevalence' of the disease in his hospital emergency – another term, which may be used is pretest probability of the disease in the population served by his emergency and suspected to have appendicitis. One should be cautious in not confusing this use of the term prevalence to how the epidemiologists define 'prevalence' – usually in the sense of community prevalence. To avoid the confusion, I prefer to use the term pretest probability (of disease).]

He tried to organise CT abdomen for all suspected cases of acute appendicitis but it did not materialise. However, he met an ultrasonographer, who sought employment claiming that he can do ultrasound test on demand and predict very well the state of inflamed versus normal appendix. The chairman employed him for 1 year on the condition that he will assess his performance in the first 200 cases of suspected acute appendicitis and then decide his future contracts. During this period, the existing policy of emergency appendectomy based on clinical diagnosis will continue. He also decided to keep his report confidential during this period.

He asked one resident to collect all his reports, keep the positives and negatives separately and in the end tally with the pathology report to tell him how often the ultrasonographically positive predictions were correct and how often the negative predictions were correct. One year passed by. The resident prepared a report which reads like this (see Table 7.5): Mr. X (US) reported 28 positive (i.e. predicted to have appendicitis), of which 25 turned out to be correct (means to have the disease), i.e. 89 %, and of 172 reported negative (predicted to have no appendicitis) 157 turned out to be correct (not to have the disease), i.e. 91 %. The chairman was pleased. He noted that if US test is positive, the probability of disease present is 25/28, i.e. 89 %, and if the test is negative, the probability of disease present is 15/172, i.e. 9 %. From a pretest probability of (disease present) 20 %, positive test result takes it to 89 % and a negative test result takes it to 9 %. Note that these are posttest probabilities of disease present. Posttest probability of 'disease absent' if the test is positive will be 11 %, and it would be 91 % if the test were negative. [Posttest probability of 'the disease absent' if the test is negative is also called 'negative predictive value'.] He concluded that the US test results are likely to be valuable, more so in reducing the unnecessary appendectomies. He was particularly pleased with correctness of the negative predictions, and he thought it will be valuable because they were very correct. This he called 'negative prediction correctness' but method experts have termed it 'negative predictive value'. So what is negative predictive value (NPV). It is the correctness of negative test results (or negative predictions). Similarly, he called the 'correctness of positive test results' (positive prediction correctness) – method experts term it 'positive predictive value (PPV)'.

Table 7.6 Definition of sensitivity, specificity and predictive values

Correctness (%) of test result	In test (predicted) positive (T+)	Positive predictive value
	In test (predicted) negative (T−)	Negative predictive value
	In (picking up) diseased (D+)	Sensitivity
	In (picking up) non-diseased (D−)	Specificity

The chairman decided to take him on permanent basis, but in the mean time, he (the chairman) had accepted a job in a paediatric centre. He decided to employ him in the paediatric centre. One day, in a dinner party, he was narrating the whole story to the pathology chairman and told him how impressed he was with the ultrasonographer, and he is going to employ him in the paediatric centre. The pathologist listened to him with interest and said, 'That's interesting but be careful. His prediction accuracy will not be as good as this in the paediatric centre'. The surgeon asked, 'Why?' The pathologist said, 'Because positive prediction correctness (or PPV) and the negative prediction correctness (or NPV) depend on the frequency of disease in the population. As acute appendicitis is more prevalent in the children, the correctness of negative prediction is likely to change.' The surgeon asked, 'how can we find that out?' The pathologist said, 'you need to find out the pickup rate of the US test (pickup rate) for the inflamed (diseased) appendix and for the normal (non-diseased) ones. You send your resident to me with all the data and I will show him. He counted the total no. of diseased appendices (40) and also how many the US had picked up. Twenty-five out of 40 were picked up. Similarly of the non-diseased ones (172), only 157 were picked up'. He said, 'the correct pickup rate (%) of "diseased" is called sensitivity, and the correct pickup rate of "non-diseased" is called specificity'. Thus, sensitivity is 62 % and specificity is 91 % (Table 7.6). In other words,

How often the +ve test result is correct? = +ve predictive value
How often the –ve test result is correct?=–ve predictive value
How often the test result is correct in 'diseased'?=sensitivity
How often the test result is correct in 'non-diseased'?=specificity

It is the sensitivity and specificity which remain relatively stable (means 'unchanged') across populations, not the predictive values (correctness). Accepting this notion, you can see that the same test has different predictive correctness in a different population with different frequency of disease.

Therefore, to determine how well the test will perform in a new setting, you need to know the prevalence (pretest probability) of the condition or disease and apply the sensitivity and specificity. Then recalculate the posttest probabilities (predictive values). [A short-cut method is to use likelihood ratio and a nomogram to determine posttest probability of the 'disease present' from pretest probability; see the next section.]

Therefore, if the pretest probability in the new setting is, say, 80 %, there will be 160 patients with the disease. Sixty-two per cent of this will be picked up, i.e. 99 and 61 will not be. Similarly of the 'non-diseased' 40 cases, 91 %, i.e. 39, will be

Table 7.7 Disease

		Disease by 'gold standard'		
		Present	Absent	Total
US	+	99	1	100
	–	61	39	100
	Total	160	40	200

picked up and one will not be. The figures will look like Table 7.7. Now, you can see that of 100 negative test results, only 39 are true negative, i.e. the US is missing a lot of patients with appendicitis and thus creating a room for disaster. The impression the ultrasonographer created in one setting is not valid for another setting. The chairman quietly retracted his decision.

So, what is the lesson? Always keep your practice setting (pretest probability) in mind while accepting a diagnostic test characteristics and recalculate the performance of the test (posttest probability) for your setting or patient and decide whether the test is good enough or not. The properties of the test, which you can transport from one setting to the other, are sensitivity, specificity or likelihood ratio (see Chap. 8).

To summarise, there are many ways to describe the performance of a diagnostic test or its results: sensitivity–specificity, predictive values and likelihood ratio. Because there are variations in the pretest probability (prevalence) of a disease, the posttest probabilities or predictive values cannot be taken from a study and applied to a patient or practice. Sensitivity, specificity or likelihood ratio is rather more stable across settings and hence can be taken from a study and applied to your practice or patient, but still what you will need to determine is the posttest probability for a given test result, keeping in mind the relevant pretest probability. There are theoretically four posttest probabilities, but only two are enough to predict the other two. It is useful to clearly keep in mind probability that positive predictive value is the posttest probability of disease present (D+) when the test result is positive, whereas negative predictive value is the posttest probability of disease absent (D–) when the test result is negative. In practice, we usually refer only to the posttest probability of disease present (D+).

Further Reading

Guyatt G, Rennie D, editors. User's guides to the medical literature: a manual for evidence-based clinical practice. Chicago: AMA Press; 2002. (www.ama-assn.org).

Hlatky MA, Pryor DB, Harrell FE. Factors affecting sensitivity and specificity of exercise electrocardiography. Am J Med. 1984;77:64–71.

Sox HC, Hickam DH, Marton KI, et al. Using the patient's history to estimate the probability of coronary artery disease: a comparison of primary care and referral practices. Am J Med. 1990;89:7–14.

Chapter 8
Diagnostic Test: Validity Appraisal

Validity Assessment (Is the Information Valid?)

Validity is the extent to which the data are free from bias. The bias can occur in the selection of sample or measurement; therefore, you must ask whether:

1. Selection bias was avoided (Was the sample selection appropriate?)
   (a) Appropriate spectrums of patients in whom there is a need for a new diagnostic test (or new diagnostic approach)?
   (b) Selected in unbiased way (e.g. consecutive cases)?
2. Measurement bias was avoided:
   (a) Was there a comparison with an appropriate gold standard?
   (b) Blinded measurement: where those doing or reporting the 'gold standard' unaware of the test result and vice versa?
   (c) No missing data: did everyone who got the test also had the gold standard [no verification bias]?

Q.1. Was the Sample Selection Appropriate?

(a) Appropriate spectrum of patients in whom there is a need for a new diagnostic test (or approach)?

You need a new diagnostic test to distinguish a disease (early as well as late) from other diseases with similar symptoms.

(b) Selected in unbiased way: consecutive patients fulfilling the entry criteria, with symptoms and signs common to both cases and non-cases ought to be included in the study.

DOI 10.1007/978-81-322-0831-0_8,

1A. Why do we ask this question?
There are many studies that include florid cases and asymptomatic volunteers. Such studies cannot tell you whether the test is useful. Probably you do not need a test to distinguish florid cases from normal people. Do you need a test to distinguish morbid obesity from normal weight. Probably not. They will be obvious to your eyes. You need to know the performance of the test in patients with diseases commonly confused with the disease you want to diagnose (also called 'target disorder'). However, you will come across many studies with florid cases and normal controls. Such studies can tell you whether the test is *useless*. If the test cannot perform as well as your eyeballs, then obviously the test is useless. Investigators often carry out such studies at some stages of development of the test. Such studies cannot tell you the performance of the test in clinical practice.

1B. How do we answer the question?
Read the methods section of the paper to find out what criteria were used for inclusion of patients in the study. Determine whether the patients so included represent (a) the disease spectrum in whom a new test is needed and also (b) the diseases commonly confused with the disease to be diagnosed (target disorder).

1C. How do we interpret the answer?
If there was only one set of eligibility (entry) criteria and it covered both cases and non-cases, then the patients are likely to suffer from commonly confused diseases. Sometimes, authors do not mention entry criteria but present the criteria for final diagnoses of cases and non-cases. In such papers, you have to decide whether in clinical practice, there is confusion between the cases and non-cases and whether there is a need for a test to distinguish them from one another.

Q.2. Was There a Comparison with an Appropriate Gold Standard?

An appropriate gold standard is the one which is 'error-free' and independent (distinct or separate) from the test under evaluation.

2A. Why do we ask this question?
The only way to evaluate the correctness of the results of the test under evaluation is to compare with something, which is never wrong. This something is called the reference standard or gold standard. This means that the gold standard is never false positive or false negative. It is 100 % sensitive and 100 % specific. However, such an ideal 'gold standard' is hardly ever available. You may have to accept something less than ideal as a reasonable gold standard. The purpose of the gold standard is to tell you the truth – did the patients have the disease or not, when the test was performed. Sometimes authors use more than one 'gold standard' to know whether the patients at the time of testing had the disease or not. For example, if you are evaluating exercise electrocardiography, you may use coronary angiography for exercise test positives and only 'follow-up' for exercise test negatives. If in 5-year follow-up,

they do not develop any symptom suggestive of coronary artery disease, you may conclude that they did not have the disease at the time of exercise test, and hence, the test was true negative.

One way the gold standard may go wrong is if the test is a part of it. For example, if you are evaluating cardiac enzymes for diagnosing myocardial infarction and you use the WHO criteria as the gold standard, which contains cardiac enzymes as its component, then there is a problem. Even when cardiac enzymes are not right, you may take them as right because the WHO criteria include them. Such a gold standard is not taken as 'independent' or distinct (separate) from the test. Whenever this happens, you get overoptimistic results for the test. Therefore, you need to ask whether the gold standard is independent of the test. Example of independent gold standard will be technetium scan for acute myocardial infarction, because it does not depend on cardiac enzymes for diagnosis of MI. Similarly in comparison of CT and MR for brain lesion, MR is independent of CT.

2B. How do we answer the question?
You need to carefully read and find out what gold standard (s) is (or are) used in the paper. From your knowledge of the subject, decide whether it (they) is (are) reasonable and whether they are independent of the test result.

2C. How do we interpret the answer?
If the gold standard is (are) not reasonable, then the results cannot be trusted. There will be overestimation or underestimation of the test properties. If the gold standard is not independent of the test result, i.e. test is a part of the gold standard, there will be overestimation of the test sensitivity and specificity. The extent of this overestimation depends on the degree of overlap (dependence) between the test result and the gold standard.

Q.3. Were Those Doing or Reporting the 'Gold Standard' Unaware of the Test Result and Vice Versa?

The test is the one under evaluation, and its correctness is being determined by comparison with the 'gold standard', which gives the definitive diagnosis.

3A. Why do we ask this question?
As clinicians, you are aware that once clinicians know the chest CT finding of pleural fluid, they start finding decreased breath sounds on auscultation; if ultrasound shows a stone in the kidney, they find a corresponding radio-opaque shadow in the plain x-ray abdomen.

Similarly, a pathologist interpreting the bone marrow biopsy may overinterpret if they know that the patient had Bence–Jones protein in urine or M-spike in serum electrophoresis. Thus, knowledge of a test result may introduce conscious or subconscious bias in the interpretation of gold standard and vice versa.

Sometimes, this question is not relevant, for example, if the gold standard result comes only after the test result or both are free from subjective errors.

3B. How do we answer the question?
The authors of the paper may write in the methods section that those doing the gold standard or the test were unaware of the results of the other. If they don't write, you have to determine from reading the methods whether those doing the test can know the results of the gold standard or those doing/reporting the gold standard could introduce conscious or subconscious bias in the result if they know the test result.

3C. How do we interpret the answer?
If there is possibility of bias due to knowledge of the test results in reporting the gold standard or vice versa, the validity of the study is compromised. The extent of compromise depends on the degree of bias, which you have to estimate from your knowledge of the condition and tests.

Q.4. Did Everyone Who Got the Test Also Had the Gold Standard (No Verification Bias)?

The gold standard is done to verify the results of the test under evaluation. By comparing the two results, we know the true positives, false positives, true negatives and false negatives of the test. Ideally, all patients should have both the test and the gold standard.

4A. Why do we ask this question?
Gold standard tests are often invasive and/or expensive. Clinicians are reluctant to perform the gold standard, when test results under evaluation are negative. For example, if you are evaluating exercise electrocardiography, you may not like to do coronary angiographies in those who are exercise test negative. Similarly, if ventilation perfusion scans are negatives, you may not like to do pulmonary angiographies, which is the 'gold standard' for pulmonary embolism.

But then how do you verify the negative test results? They may be false negatives. Some investigators follow up the patients for a period of time (without specific treatment). If the patients do not develop direct or indirect features of the disease, they are taken as true negatives, otherwise as false negatives. If there is no follow-up or any other way to verify the negatives, the study suffers from verification bias (there are some statistical methods to correct for this bias, but they are beyond the scope of this book).

4B. How do we answer the question?
The results section of the paper gives you the number of patients who underwent the test and the gold standard. If all those undergoing the test were subjected to the gold standard, there is no problem. More than one gold standard may be used, for example, angiographies and follow-up. If both are acceptable, again there is no problem. If some patients had not undergone the gold standard test and were not followed up or subjected to another gold standard, there may be a problem. You need to find out whether the results are still valid (see below).

4C. How do we interpret the answer?
One way to find out whether the results are still valid is as follows:
The number of patients, negative on the test but no gold standard (means no verification), may be assumed to be false negative, and the test characteristics may be recalculated. If they are still acceptable, then the results may be taken as valid, in spite of verification bias. However, if test characteristics become unacceptable, then the validity of the results is compromised.

The above false-negative assumption is extreme and unlikely to be true, but if a study passes this extreme assumption, then the results are strong. Otherwise, you don't know whether the results are valid or not. You doubt the validity of the results.

Results Assessment: What Is the Information?

In this section, you need to know whether any of the test results are likely to help in ruling in or ruling out the disease of interest, detailed in the next chapter (see Chap. 9).

Applicability Assessment

Is the Test Available and Reproducible in My Clinical Setting?

The test availability includes not only the equipment and reagents required for the test but also the human resource (e.g. technicians and experts). If they are available, the next question is, can they reproduce the same result when the test is repeated in stable patients?

Are Patients in My Practice Similar to Those in the Study?

You need to think whether the disease severity and the conditions in differential diagnosis of the disease in your practice are similar to those in the study. Otherwise, the test parameters (sensitivity, specificity, likelihood ratio [LR]) may not strictly apply, though roughly you can still use them.

Will the Results Change My Management?

This is a very important question. You know the pretest probability in your setting. You know the LRs of the test results, and you determine the posttest probabilities and then ask whether these are likely to change your decision. If the test results, even if one, is likely to change your management, then the test is helpful.

Will Your Patients Be Better Off as a Result of the Test?

It is not enough to say that the test results will change your management. What you need to think is whether as a result of this changed management, your patients are likely to be better off. Better off may mean better health, earlier discharge to home, less inconvenience, early return to work and even less expenses. Then whatever benefit comes, is it worth the costs and risk of the test?

Application

As usual, first assess the patients with history and physical examination and determine the pretest probability of the disease, then do the diagnostic test and get the result. The likelihood ratio associated with this result will take you from pretest probability to posttest probability. Based on this, take a decision whether to treat and do another test or rule out this possibility. If ruled out, consider other diagnostic tests (see example in Chap. 12).

Further Reading

Bates SE. Clinical applications of serum tumor markers. Ann Intern Med. 1991;115:623–38.

Begg CB, Greenes RA. Assessment of diagnostic tests when disease verification is subject to selection bias. Biometrics. 1983;39:207–15.

Catalona WJ, et al. Measurement of prostate-specific antigen in serum as a screening test for prostate cancer. N Engl J Med. 1991;324:1156–61.

Choi BC. Sensitivity and specificity of a single diagnostic test in the presence of work-up bias. J Clin Epidemiol. 1992;45:581–6.

Fletcher RH. Carcinoembryonic antigen. Ann Intern Med. 1986;104:66–73.

Gray R, Begg CB, Greenes RA. Construction of receiver operating characteristic curves when disease verification is subject to selection bias. Med Decis Making. 1984;4:151–64.

Grinder PF, Mayewski RJ, Mushlin AI, Greenland P. Selection and interpretation of diagnostic tests and procedure. Principles and applications. Ann Intern Med. 1981;94:557–600.

Guyatt GH, Tugwell PX, Feeny DH, Haynes RB, Drummond M. A framework for clinical evaluation of diagnostic technologies. CMAJ. 1986;134:587–94.

Guyatt G, Rennie D, editors. User's guides to the medical literature: a manual for evidence-based clinical practice. Chicago: AMA Press; 2002. www.ama-assn.org.

Lijmer JG, Mol BW, Heisterkamp S, et al. Empirical evidence of design-related bias in studies of diagnostic tests. JAMA. 1999;282:1061–6.

Ransohoff DF, Feinstein AR. Problems of spectrum and bias in evaluating the efficacy of diagnostic tests. N Engl J Med. 1978;299:926–30.

Sheps SB, Schechter MT. The assessment of diagnostic tests. A survey of current medical research. JAMA. 1984;104:60–6.

Voss JD. Prostate cancer, screening, and prostate-specific antigen: promise or peril? J Gen Intern Med. 1994;9:468–74.

Wasson JH, Sox Jr HC, Neff RK, Goldman L. Clinical prediction rules, applications and methodological standards. N Engl J Med. 1985;313:793–9.

Chapter 9
Diagnostic Test: Critical Appraisal – Part 2 (Interpreting Results)

Two-Level (Dichotomous) Test Results

Tests with Positive/Negative Results: In the dichotomous situation, we usually use two measures of validity (sensitivity and specificity). You can use only likelihood ratio (see later). Validity refers to the degree of correctness of results. 'Sensitivity' and 'specificity' are measures of validity.

Sensitivity is the proportion (or probability) of correct (positive) result in those with disease. This may also be called *'true positivity'* if positivity is taken to indicate presence of disease or 'true positive rate' (but actually this is a proportion, not a rate). This is determined by dividing the number of true positive by the number with disease in the study:

$$\text{Sensitivity} = \frac{\text{No. of true positives}}{\text{No. of subjects with the disease}} \tag{9.1}$$

Specificity is the proportion (or probability) of correct (negative) result in those without disease. If the correct result in those without disease is taken as 'negative', then specificity may also be called *'true negativity'* or 'true negative rate'. This is determined by dividing the number of true negatives by the number without the disease in the study, i.e.

$$\text{Specificity} = \frac{\text{No. of true negatives}}{\text{No. of subjects without the disease}} \tag{9.2}$$

It is desirable to have high sensitivity as well as high specificity. But often, a test is highly sensitive but not highly specific and vice versa. How can we deal with such situations? Well, a highly sensitive test, even if not very specific, can help to 'rule out' a disease, if it turns out to be 'negative'. To remember this, we use the mnemonic 'SnNOUT'. A highly sensitive (Sn) test, if negative (N), rules OUT the disease.

K. Prasad, *Fundamentals of Evidence-Based Medicine*,
DOI 10.1007/978-81-322-0831-0_9, © Springer India 2013

High sensitivity in this context is usually taken as between 0.95 (95 %) and 100 %, depending on the disease under consideration.

Similarly a highly specific test, even if not highly sensitive, can help to 'rule in' a disease, if it turns out to be 'positive'. To remember this, we use the mnemonic 'SpPIN'. A highly specific (Sp) test, if positive (P), rules IN the disease. High specificity, in this context, is usually taken as 0.95 (95 %) or above.

What do we do if a test is neither 95 % sensitive nor 95 % specific, but 80 % sensitive and 85 % specific? How do we assess its value? How do we respond if a highly sensitive test is positive or a highly specific test is negative? Let us remember that a test is valuable if it significantly changes the probability of a disease (from pretest to posttest). What do we mean by 'significantly'? 'Significant' change here means the change which prompts a decision to treat or do another (probably more invasive) test (from indecisive stage). Now, this depends on what the pretest probability is. If pretest probability is 80 %, then the test with 80 % sensitivity and 85 % specificity, when positive, yields a posttest probability of 95 %. This will nearly always prompt initiation of treatment. Therefore, the test is valuable.

How do we know whether (and how much) a test result will change the pretest probability? For this we need a test parameter called likelihood ratio.

Likelihood Ratio

Likelihood ratio is a link between pretest probabilities and posttest probabilities. It takes you from one to the other (pre to post).

Likelihood ratio (LR) is a ratio of two likelihoods: one in diseased (those with the disease of interest) and the other in non-diseased (non-diseased does not necessarily mean healthy; it means those without the disease of interest). LR tells us how many times more (or less) often a test result is seen among those with the disease as compared to those without the disease. To determine this, we obviously need a ratio which compares likelihood of a test result among those with the disease compared with those without the disease. In other words,

$$\text{LR} = \frac{\text{Likelihood of a test result in those with disease (the disease present)}}{\text{Likelihood of the same result in those without the disease (the disease absent)}}$$

If we know this, it is easy to find the posttest probability either using a nomogram or a formula. The nomogram prepared by Fagan [1] has three vertical lines. You need to select one point corresponding to the pretest probability and the second corresponding to the likelihood ratio of the test result on the appropriate lines of the nomogram. If you join these two lines and extend it to meet the rightmost line of the nomogram, the meeting point gives you the posttest probability of the disease with the given test result. You can also use the following formula to determine posttest probability from pretest probability and likelihood ratio:

$$\text{Post-test probability} = \frac{\text{Pre-test probability} \times \text{LR}}{1 + \text{Pre-test probability (LR} - 1)} \tag{9.3}$$

For example, let us consider the study by Guyatt et al. [2] for diagnosis of iron-deficiency anaemia in the elderly. Let us ask how good is serum ferritin level in diagnosis of iron-deficiency anaemia in the elderly. Guyatt et al. included 235 consecutive elderly patients with anaemia in the study. Serum ferritin and bone marrow aspiration results (gold standard) were obtained in all the patients. The results are presented in Table 9.1.

As you see, serum ferritin results have been grouped into four subgroups. A subgroup is called 'stratum' (plural strata). We can say the serum ferritin results are presented in four strata. Now, let us calculate LRs. LR is always for a test result (not for a test). Since there are four strata of test results, we will calculate an LR for each stratum separately (stratum-specific LR). Let us recap the formula for LR:

$$\begin{aligned}\text{LR of a test result} &= \frac{\text{Likelihood of the result in 'diseased'}}{\text{Likelihood of the same result in 'non-diseased'}} \\ &= \frac{\text{\% of diseased having the test result}}{\text{\% of non-diseased having the same test result.}}\end{aligned}$$

Stratum-specific likelihood ratios (LR) for serum ferritin level:

$$\text{LR for} \leq 18\ \mu\text{g/L} = \frac{\text{\% of diseased having} \leq 18\ \mu\text{g/L}}{\text{\% of non-diseased having} \leq 18\ \mu\text{g/L}}$$

Total no. of 'disease' are 85.
No. of 'diseased' having ≤18 μg/L = 47.

$$\text{Therefore, \% of diseased having} \leq 18\ \mu\text{g/L} = \frac{47}{85} \times 100$$

Total no. of 'non-diseased' (not iron deficient) = 150.
No. of 'non-diseased' (Not iron deficient) having ≤18 μg/L = 2.

Table 9.1 Results of a study of iron deficiency anaemia: serum ferritin vs bone marrow (gold standard)

	Bone marrow result	
Serum ferritin level (μg/L)	Iron deficient	Not iron deficient
≤18	47	2
>18–45	23	13
>45–100	7	27
>100	8	108
Total	85	150

$$\text{Therefore, \% of non-diseased having} \le 18\,\mu g/L = \frac{2}{150} \times 100$$

$$\text{LR for} \le 18\,\mu g/L = \frac{\frac{47}{85} \times 100}{\frac{2}{150} \times 100} = 41.5$$

$$\text{LR for} > 18-45 = \frac{\frac{23}{85} \times 100}{\frac{13}{150} \times 100} = 3.1$$

$$\text{LR for} > 45-100 = \frac{\frac{7}{85} \times 100}{\frac{27}{150} \times 100} = 0.46$$

$$\text{LR for} > 100 = \frac{\frac{8}{85} \times 100}{\frac{108}{150} \times 100} = 0.13$$

Now, the question is how will you interpret them.

Interpretation of LR: General

What do LRs mean? The LRs indicate by how much a given diagnostic test result will raise or lower the pretest probability of the 'disease' under consideration.

LR of 1.0 = (means) posttest probability of the disease is exactly the same as its pretest probability.
LR of >1.0 increases the posttest probability of the 'disease'; the higher the LR, the greater is the increase.
LR of <1.0 decreases the posttest probability of the disease; the smaller the LR, the greater is the decrease.

LR of 10,000 rules in the disease, even if pretest probability is <1 %. Similarly LR of 0.0001 rules out the disease, even if pretest probability is 99 %.

A general rough guide to interpret LRs is as follows:

- LRs of >10 or <0.1 often generate substantial changes from pre- to posttest probability, so much so that the next step is clear.
- LRs of 5–10 and 0.1–0.2 generate moderate and usually conclusive changes from pre- to posttest probability.
- LRs of 2–5 and 0.5–0.2 generate small but rarely important changes from pre- to posttest probability.
- LRs of 1–2 and 0.5–1 generate practically no important changes from pre- to posttest probability.

Interpretation of LR: Specific

When it comes to a specific setting or a specific patient, a given LR is useful if it helps in decision-making; in other words, it changes the management strategy.

Two things are necessary:

1. You need to have a rough estimate of pretest probability.
2. You need to have a threshold (have a decision point in) posttest probability beyond which you will take a decision to take the next step (do a more invasive test, treat, admit or discharge).

For the given estimate of your pretest probability and the reported LR of the test result, find the posttest probability. If this is beyond the threshold, it means the LR is helpful (e.g. see below).

Connection Between Sensitivity, Specificity and the Likelihood Ratio

The question is: Is there any connection between sensitivity, specificity and the likelihood ratio? The answer is clearly yes. We can interpret and use tests with dichotomous results without referring to their sensitivity and specificity, but there is clearly a connection between the two, as shown below.

Let us use our usual formula for LR for a test result:

$$= \frac{\text{\% of diseased having the result}}{\text{\% of non-diseased having the result}}$$

When the result is positive, the formula becomes

$$\text{LR for 'positive' test result (LR+)} = \frac{\text{\% of diseased having + result}}{\text{\% of non-diseased having a + result}} = \frac{\text{\% true + ve}}{\text{\% False + ve}} = \frac{\text{Sensitivity (\%)}}{100 - \text{Specificity (\%)}},$$

$$\text{In decimals} = \frac{\text{Sensitivity}}{1 - \text{Specificity}}$$

$$\text{LR for 'negative' test result (LR−)} = \frac{\text{\% of diseased having − ve result}}{\text{\% of non-diseased having a − ve result}} = \frac{\text{\% False − ve}}{\text{\% True − ve}} = \frac{100 - \text{Sensitivity \%}}{\text{Specificity \%}},$$

$$\text{In decimals} = \frac{1 - \text{Sensitivity}}{\text{Specificity}}$$

Therefore, for a sensitivity of 80 % and specificity of 85 %, LR will be 80/15 = 5.3. With a pretest probability of 80 % (0.8), the posttest probability of disease with positive test result using formula (9.3) will be 95.5 %. Thus, you can see that the test can be used to 'rule in' the disease even with sensitivity of 80 % and specificity of 85 %, provided pretest probability is 80 %.

The following table (Table 9.2) gives the required likelihood ratios for ruling in or ruling out a disease when the pretest probability is known. For example, if the pretest probability is 30 %, then for posttest probability of 95 %, the LR of a given test result should be 44, and for posttest probability of 5 %, the likelihood ratio of the given test result should be 0.12. Thus, this table will help you to interpret the ability of a given likelihood ratio to rule in or rule out disease with certain pretest probability.

Sometimes clinicians have to decide a management strategy for their patients based on probabilities of the disease that are <95 or 99 %. For example, a patient presenting to the emergency room with chest pain needs to be assessed and a decision has to be made whether to admit the patient to the coronary care unit. Even if the posttest probability of acute myocardial infarction (AMI) is 20 %, nearly all clinicians would like to admit him to the coronary care unit and observe for at least 48 h

Table 9.2 Likelihood ratios to rule in/out the disease

	LR to rule in		LR to rule out		
Pretest probability	Posttest probability 95 %	Posttest probability 99 %	Posttest probability 0.5 %	Posttest probability 1 %	Posttest probability 5 %
0.01	1881	9801	–	1	–
0.05	361	1881	0.09	0.19	1
0.1	171	891	0.05	0.09	0.47
0.2	76	396	0.02	0.04	0.21
0.3	44	231	0.01	0.02	0.12
0.4	29	149	0.007	0.015	0.07
0.5	19	99	0.005	0.01	0.05
0.6	13	66	0.003	0.007	0.03
0.7	8	42	0.002	0.004	0.02
0.8	5	25	0.001	0.002	0.01
0.9	2	11	0.0006	0.001	0.005

to rule in or rule out AMI. We, therefore, need to know whether a given likelihood ratio of a test result can give us a posttest probability of 20 %. The following table (Table 9.3) gives the required likelihood ratios to revise pretest probabilities in the range of 1–90 % to posttest probabilities in the range from 1 to 99 %. To use this table, start with your estimate of pretest probability of a disease, then determine the likelihood ratio associated with test result and then find out where does this LR fall in the row of your pretest probability. The top row corresponding to the place of LR will give you the posttest probability or the figures between which this is likely to fall.

Where do you Get the Pretest Probabilities from?

It comes from your experience, from a study or from your hospital data. If your hospital keeps the data of frequency of diagnoses, it might be a good source. If you take it from a study, you need to check how relevant are its results for your practice. Most commonly, you will have to depend on your own experience of having seen such diseases. Moreover, the more risk factors, signs and symptoms are present in a case, the more is the pretest probability.

Table 9.3 Likelihood ratios to revise given pretest probabilities to various posttest probabilities

Pretest	Posttest probabilities											
probabilities	1 %	5 %	10 %	20 %	30 %	40 %	50 %	60 %	70 %	80 %	90 %	95 %	99 %
0.01	1	5.21	11	24.75	42.43	66	99	148.5	231.	396	891	1881	9801
0.05	0.19	1	2.11	4.75	21	32.67	49	73.5	114.33	196	441	361	1881
0.1	0.091	0.47	1	2.25	3.86	6	9	13.5	21	36	81	171	891
0.2	0.04	0.21	0.44	1	1.71	2.67	4	6	9.33	16	36	76	396
0.3	0.02	0.12	0.26	0.58	1	1.56	2.33	3.5	5.44	9.33	21	44	231
0.4	0.02	0.08	0.17	0.38	0.64	1	1.5	2.25	3.5	6	13.5	29	149
0.5	0.01	0.05	0.11	0.25	0.43	0.67	1	1.5	2.33	4	9	19	99
0.6	0.007	0.04	0.07	0.17	0.27	0.44	0.67	1	1.56	2.67	6	13	66
0.7	0.004	0.023	0.05	0.10	0.18	0.27	0.43	0.64	1	1.71	3.86	8	42
0.8	0.003	0.013	0.03	0.06	0.11	0.17	0.25	0.38	0.58	1	2.25	5	25
0.9	0.001	0.006	0.01	0.02	0.05	0.07	0.11	0.17	0.26	0.44	1	2	11

Conclusion

The above discussion describes all the necessary parameters to evaluate a diagnostic test. The present trend is to move towards likelihood ratio, but the commonly known parameters sensitivity and specificity should be understood as well. This chapter helps you to understand these concepts.

References

1. Fagan TJ. Nomogram for Bayes's theorem. N Engl J Med. 1975;293:257.
2. Guyatt GH, Oxman AD, Ali M, Willan A, McIlroy W, Patterson C. Laboratory diagnosis of iron-deficiency anemia: an overview. J Gen Intern Med. 1992;7:145–53.

Further Reading

Cebul RD, Beck LH. Teaching clinical decision-making. New York: Praeger; 1985.

Department of Clinical Epidemiology and Biostatistics, McMaster University. Interpretation of diagnostic data. V. How to do it with simple math. Can Med Assoc J. 1983;129-22-29.

Diamond GA, Forrester JS. Analysis of probability as an aid in the clinical diagnosis of coronary artery disease. N Engl J Med. 1979;300:1350–8.

Fletcher RH. Carcinoembryonic antigen. Ann Intern Med. 1986;104:66–73.

Grinder PF, Mayewski RJ, Mushlin AI, Greenland P. Selection and interpretation of diagnostic tests and procedure. Principles and applications. Ann Intern Med. 1981;94:557–600.

Guyatt G, Rennie D, editors. User's guides to the medical literature: a manual for evidence-based clinical practice. Chicago: AMA Press; 2002. (www.ama-assn.org).

Hlatky MA, Pryor DB, Harrell FE. Factors affecting sensitivity and specificity of exercise electrocardiography. Am J Med. 1984;77:64–71.

The PIOPED Investigators. Value of the ventilation/perfusion scan in acute pulmonary embolism. Results of the prospective investigation of pulmonary embolism diagnosis (PIOPED). JAMA. 1990;263:2753–9.

Wasson JH, Sox Jr HC, Neff RK, Goldman L. Clinical prediction rules, applications and methodological standards. N Engl J Med. 1985;313:793–9.

Chapter 10
Systematic Review and Meta-analysis: Fundamental Concepts

Origin of the Term 'Meta-analysis'

The term 'meta-analysis' was first used by Gene Glass in his presidential address to the American Educational Research Association in 1976. He distinguished it from primary analysis (analysis of original data in a research study, usually carried out under the direction of those who designed the study) and secondary analysis (reanalysis of the data with better statistical techniques usually carried out by someone not involved in the design of the original study). Meta-analysis, according to Glass, is a statistical analysis of summary results of individual studies for the purpose of integrating the findings. It may be noted, however, that the idea of combining results from separate studies can be traced to 1904 when Pearson first used data pooling. In 1932, Sir Ronald Fisher reported on combining *P* values. Gene Glass advanced the field by making original and groundbreaking contributions.

Scope of Meta-analysis

In recent years, the term 'meta-analysis' has been used in a broad sense, and its scope has also enlarged. Meta-analysis is being used in almost all branches of science including meteorology, agriculture, psychology, nuclear physics and, of course, medicine.

In medicine, meta-analyses may be done on surveys, diagnostic, prognostic or a etiologic studies, but most of meta-analyses to date evaluate treatment studies. The following description applies largely to meta-analysis of treatment studies.

What Is Meta-analysis?

Simply said, meta-analysis is a study of studies. However, different people use the term to mean different things. Most experts use the term to refer to the statistical

K. Prasad, *Fundamentals of Evidence-Based Medicine*,
DOI 10.1007/978-81-322-0831-0_10, © Springer India 2013

(quantitative) combination of results from two or more studies addressing the same research question. Others use it to refer to systematic reviews. To understand the strengths and limitations of meta-analysis, we need to know how it differs from 'traditional' and 'systematic' reviews.

Need for Reviews

We are witnessing unprecedented information explosion. More than 1,000,000 articles are published each year in more than 20,000 journals. It is humanly impossible to read through all the articles published in any given field. Therefore, we need concise summaries of the literature, after separating the insignificant and unsound from salient and crucial. Such summaries are found in review articles in journals.

Traditional (Narrative) Reviews: What Is It?

Students, residents as well as experts often look for review articles. When residents have to present seminars or journal clubs, when experts have to deliver lectures or talks or write a chapter in a book and when practitioners want to update their knowledge and learn about new treatments or diagnostic tests, they go through the recent issues of some reputed journals in the field and look for a relevant review article. Most journals publish review articles regularly.

How are these articles written? Most often, an expert on the topic is invited or motivated to write a review article. He collects as many articles on the topic as he can find. He goes through them with varying interest. Then, he summarises the findings in his own writing style. More often than not, he has his own preconceptions about the topic (based on his own publications) that have varying influence on what he writes. The articles undergo editorial review before being published in the journals. Such review articles are sometimes referred to as 'traditional reviews'. They may be defined as review articles written by one or more experts based on a convenience sample of studies with no description of the underlying methodology.

Strengths of Traditional Reviews

They cover a wide range of issues on a topic in a concise manner. Often, articles on a clinical issue provide a succinct summary of basic sciences in relation to the topic. Articles on a disease like hepatitis might cover epidemiology, aetiology, pathogenesis, pathology, natural history and treatment. The treatment part may cover all the available drug or surgical treatment.

Limitations of Traditional Reviews

The traditional review articles (also called 'narrative' reviews) have served the summarising function, but they usually have one or more of the following limitations.

1. *Lack of explicit methodology*:
   Traditional review articles usually do not carry any 'methods' section. The reader is left uncertain whether a comprehensive search of relevant papers has been done, whether the inclusion of papers for reference has been unbiased and whether steps have been taken to limit errors in the reviewing process and that due to the primary studies.
2. *Vote-counting*:
   Often, writers of the traditional reviews resort to vote-counting. They count the number of studies in favour of an intervention and the number against. Then, they may support the side having the greater number of studies. This is fallible. They count even 'incompetent' votes. Votes are incompetent when they have errors. Errors are because of inadequacy in the quality or quantity of data. Without adequate data, authors conclude against an intervention. This is like saying, 'Absence of proof (of benefit) is the proof of absence (of benefit)', but this is not true.

   One ought to see the result of a study in view of its limitations. A small single-centre study should not be counted equal to a large multicentric one. An open non-randomised study should not be given the same weight as a randomised placebo controlled one. In other words, reviewers ought to give weight according to the quality and quantity of the data in the studies. Most traditional reviews do not do this.
3. *Over-reliance on intermediate outcomes (end points)*:
   It has been observed that many traditional reviews give undue importance to the intermediate patient outcomes. This may be misleading and, at times, dangerous. A dramatic example is the 'trial of encainide and flecainide' [1, 2]. These drugs were shown to suppress abnormal ventricular depolarisations, but in the randomised trial, the mortality was substantially higher in the patients receiving the antiarrhythmic drugs. Reviewers relying on only arrhythmia as the outcome could have erroneously concluded in favour of the drugs. The error would occur because of over-reliance on intermediate outcomes. The intermediate outcomes must be closely and strongly related to the clinically important outcomes for reviewers to consider recommending on the basis of those. Such relationships are few and far between.
4. *'Missed opportunity' to combine the results*:
   Traditional reviews often look at the individual studies separately but do not combine their results, even if they are combinable. Thus, they may miss an opportunity to arrive at clearer conclusions, which may be possible after combining the results.

   'Unity is strength' is a famous adage. By uniting (combining) the results of the individual studies, reviewers may gain strength (power), which in turn may permit clear-cut conclusions even if individual studies were inconclusive.

Systematic Reviews (SRs) Versus Meta-analysis

Definition

A systematic review may be defined as a review addressing a specific research question (on treatment, diagnosis, prognosis or aetiology) using explicit methodology of collecting, selecting and appraising studies and, whenever appropriate, synthesising their results quantitatively.

The definition indicates that the systematic review may have only qualitative or both qualitative and quantitative components. The qualitative component consists of the assessment of quality of individual studies, whereas the quantitative component is the meta-analysis.

The National Library of Medicine (NLM) of the USA has included in MEDLINE the term 'meta-analysis' as subject heading in 1989 and as publication type in 1993. It does not have systematic review as a medical subject heading or publication type. This may be one reason why the term meta-analysis is more popular.

Systematic Review but not Meta-analysis

Some experts would not use the term 'meta-analysis' for such systematic reviews, which do not contain statistical combination of the results of the studies. The combination may not be required if there is only one study, it may not be possible if the studies report different outcomes or it may not be desirable if the studies have widely varying results due to reasons such as differences in study population or intervention. Sometimes, a systematic review may conclude that there is no worthwhile study on the topic. Under such circumstances, it may not be acceptable to use the term meta-analysis but such circumstances are rare.

Meta-analysis but not Systematic Review

Sometimes, authors may not use a systematic process to search, select and appraise the studies on a given topic, yet find some convenient sample of studies and combine the results of the studies statistically and call it a meta-analysis. Technically it may be a meta-analysis, but it cannot be called a systematic review, because the process of finding, selecting or appraising the studies has not been systematic. Such meta-analysis may lead to erroneous results. They are poorly conducted meta-analyses.

Fortunately, most meta-analyses are not so poorly conducted, and also most systematic reviews do combine the results of the studies statistically. Hence, for practical purposes, most systematic reviews contain a meta-analysis, and hence the common usage of titles like 'a systematic review and meta-analysis'.

Strengths of Systematic Reviews/Meta-analysis

Good systematic reviews (SRs) have several strengths, for example:

1. *Comprehensive search strategy*:
   Good systematic reviews usually scan multiple sources of information. For example, Cochrane reviews use electronic databases, hand searching, experts, specialised registers of trials and personal contacts to retrieve relevant studies.
2. *Explicit methodology*:
   Systematic reviews are undertaken on the premise that they should be reproducible like any other scientific activity. This requires that the methods followed in conducting the review be described in such detail that allows any other reviewer to reproduce it with the same results. So, there is a 'methods' section in a systematic review explicitly describing the steps and definitions used.
3. *Emphasis on all clinically important outcomes*:
   SRs, particularly Cochrane reviews, emphasise on all clinically relevant outcomes related to efficacy, safety and tolerability of the interventions under consideration.
4. *Limiting errors*:
   SRs usually have two reviewers at all major steps to limit errors in conducting the review. Reviewers appraise the quality and quantity of data in each of the primary studies and accordingly give appropriate weights to the studies under review. This tends to limit bias in the results and improve prediction in what to expect while extrapolating the results.

The Process of a Meta-analysis: Essential Steps

Most meta-analyses include the following steps:

Steps	Process of meta-analysis
1.	Research question and a protocol
2.	Comprehensive search
3.	Selection of studies
4.	Appraisal (quality assessment) of studies
5.	Data abstraction
6.	Data analysis
	(a) Assessing combinability
	(b) Selecting the formula for combining

Step 1: Research Question and a Protocol

Meta-analysis, like any other research activity, starts with a research question. The research question specifies the population of interest, the exposure or intervention, the comparison (in certain situations) and the outcome of interest.

A protocol specifying the research question, search methods, criteria for including or excluding a study, criteria for quality assessment (appraisal) of the studies and methods of data extraction and synthesis is written. Subgroup analyses, if any, are pre-specified. Cochrane collaboration has a system of reviewing the protocol and publishing it in the Cochrane Library. The steps detailed below are then followed according to the protocol.

Step 2: Comprehensive Search

There is no way to prove that a reviewer has found all the relevant studies. One thing seems clear from empirical studies, that is, no single source is comprehensive enough. MEDLINE, arguably the best source for medical literature, does not yield all the relevant studies and what it yields is often irrelevant. For published studies, the best possible method (called 'the gold standard') is hand searching, that is, going through every article of the journals and selecting the relevant studies. [The percent (or proportion) of (relevant) studies found through MEDLINE compared to hand searching is termed 'sensitivity' of MEDLINE searching. The percent or proportion of the yield that is relevant is called 'specificity'.]

In some fields like ophthalmology, empirical studies have shown that MEDLINE yields 50 % (sensitivity) of the relevant studies that are found through hand searching of the indexed journals. This means indexing has not been good in certain fields. Also, the specificity of the yield (percent relevant) is also around 50 % in certain fields. However, hand searching is a labour-intensive process. Under the aegis of the Cochrane Collaboration, a number of volunteers are conducting hand searching of various journals and registering all controlled studies in a Central Register, which is quarterly published in the Cochrane Library.

Reviewers adopt multiple overlapping methods to ascertain the relevant studies as comprehensively as possible. Non-MEDLINE electronic databases (EMBASE, Cochrane Library, etc.) are searched. Cochrane review groups have search coordinators to maintain a specialised register of studies and find relevant studies. Reviewers display posters with list of studies in conferences and seek additional studies from subject experts. The experts often point to additional studies (published as well as unpublished). Writing to the experts can also be rewarding in this regard. Many reviewers write to the drug manufacturers to gather unpublished studies of a drug.

Cochrane reviews are meant to be updated as and when more studies (new or old) are found. Search for studies is continued even after the publication of Cochrane reviews. In this sense, search is a never-ending process. Reviewers as well as review group coordinators remain perpetually alert to find a study worthy of inclusion in the review.

Step 3: Selection of Studies

Reviewers use predefined inclusion (and exclusion) criteria to select studies for the review. The criteria refer to the study design, specific population, intervention, comparison and outcome relevant for the research question. Studies meeting the criteria are selected for the next steps.

Step 4: Appraisal (Quality Assessment) of Studies

Reviewers use explicit criteria to assess the quality of the selected studies. The criteria may vary from topic to topic to some extent but include the basic elements of credibility of randomisation, blinded outcome assessment, extent of follow-up and intention-to-treat analysis.

Some authors use scales to assess the quality of studies. There are more than 25 scales in the literature. None of them are valid and applicable to all types of studies. I believe that the reviewers should combine the basic (mentioned above) and topic-specific elements of quality to form a scale for use in the review. For example, Prasad et al. [3] added the use of CT scan for diagnosis as a topic-specific element in their meta-analysis of surgery in intracerebral haemorrhage. At least two reviewers assess the quality of the studies.

Step 5: Data Abstraction

At least two reviewers read the results of the studies and abstract data using a pre-tested data abstraction form. The data usually pertain to multiple outcomes (beneficial as well as adverse) and often to separate subgroups of patients. For dichotomous data, the data can be displayed into 2×2 tables, one for each outcome or subgroup. For continuous data, means and standard deviations are extracted for each group/subgroup of patients. Sample size of each study is also noted.

Sometimes, it is necessary to write to the authors to obtain certain data not included in the published reports.

[N.B. The above description does not apply to meta-analyses involving individual patient data (often referred to as IPD meta-analyses). In IPD meta-analyses, the files containing individual patient data are joined to form a joint file of all the data with study identifiers as a variable. The topic is beyond the scope of this book]

Step 6: Data Synthesis

This step has several sub-steps.

Sub-step 6 (a): Assessing Combinability

This involves assessing the similarity of results. Similarity of results is called 'homogeneity'. Dissimilarity is called 'heterogeneity'. The question of similarity means asking, 'Are the different studies saying (or indicating) the same thing?'. The question is approached from clinical as well as statistical angles. Clinically, reviewers judge whether the population, intervention, comparison and outcome measurements are similar enough in the various studies to justify combining the results. Here, readers may wonder whether this question is at all necessary. They may argue, when the inclusion of studies, in the first place, requires pre-specified population, intervention, comparison and outcome, they are bound to be similar. So, why does this question arise? Well, this is a matter of the level of specificity one goes up to. In inclusion criteria, reviewers may specify like this:

Population: Acute ischaemic stroke with onset within 6 h
Intervention: Thrombolytics
Comparison: Conventional treatment
Outcome: Death, full recovery

But in assessing combinability, they may ask, 'Are the studies using the same thrombolytic agent, for example, streptokinase (SK)? Should we combine studies using streptokinase with those using t-PA (tissue plasminogen activator)? The answers to these questions call for clinical judgment, involve subjectivity and are not always unanimous (incidentally, experts disagree on whether SK and t-PA studies should be combined. In such situations, combined as well as separate results of the subset of studies are presented).

Combinability may be clear on looking at the plot of the study results as point estimates and confidence intervals (CI). Look whether the point estimates are close to each other and whether the CIs are overlapping (for more details, see next chapter).

Statistical approach to this question involves asking the question: 'Assuming all studies are similar (homogeneous), what is the chance (probability) of finding the results as different or similar as we do?' If this chance is small (say, 10 or 5 %), then we reject our assumption of similarity. If the chance is more than 10 %, then we accept (sometimes wrongly – as you may think) that the studies are similar.

If both approaches support similarity, there is no problem. If there are differences, we combine both overall as well as subset of studies.

Sub-step 6(b): Selecting the Formula for Combining

After deciding to combine, we have to select from a number of different formulae. I will discuss only two: One is called 'formula of fixed effects model', and second is called 'formula of random effects model'. There are ardent supporters and critics of both among the top statisticians.

A detailed discussion is beyond the scope of this paper. Suffice it to say that if all the studies had followed the same study protocol and were conducted at the same time (contemporaneously), there would be little or no hesitation in using the fixed effects model. Investigators often use this model for combining results across centres in multicentric studies. Again, the extent to which the protocol and timing of the studies differ will determine whether one model is justified or the other. I often use both and if both approaches yield the same conclusions, I consider the conclusions are strong. If they differ, the conclusions are 'weak' and more studies or other sources of evidence (e.g. nonrandomised studies) are necessary to support the conclusions.

A rough idea about the two methods can be gained using this example. Suppose you want to conduct a research to determine whether computer-based mathematics teaching (and practice exercises) is superior to traditional (chalk and board with paper-based exercises). You arrange a workshop of ten teachers from across your country and train them how to teach math based on computer. You then give them all the necessary materials (computer, printer, software, etc.) and ask them to carry out a randomised study in their own settings with one arm of students receiving traditional and another arm receiving computer-based teaching. At the end, all students receive a math test, and you compare the two groups. Now suppose you want to do a meta-analysis of the ten studies. The question is whether you should take into account only the sample differences or also other somewhat inapparent differences. If you ignore the other unmeasured or unknown causes of the differences, you are saying that each centre had two groups and all centres are measuring the same effect except due to differences in the sample of students. This will be called fixed effects models. If you want to take into account the differences among centres (unknown or unmeasured causes), you are saying that the effects vary due to both the samples and some other factors, not known or measured. The effect is also a random variable, it's not fixed. Therefore, this approach is called random effects model. Which one do you prefer? You may favour the latter, because you know that teachers vary in their competence as regards their teaching competence and their computer literacy. But in clinical trials the situation is less clear: People argue that all studies used the same drug in the same condition in the same dosage – so the effects you get will also be the same and thus favour fixed effects model. Others argue in favour of random effects model. You may like to use my preference of using or looking for both and see if the results differ.

There is another way to conceptualise the two models. In fixed effects model, you are interested in only the given (in the above example, ten) studies and you consider them to constitute the universe, whereas in the random effects you consider the given studies as a sample from the universe. They are used to get an idea how the results would have varied had you have thousand of studies. The random effects model takes into account this variability as well as the variability due to the sample differences (for more details on this, please see Chap. 13).

Sub-step 6(c): Weight of the Studies in a Meta-analysis

The following may help you to understand the basis of weights assigned to a study in a meta-analysis with binary (dichotomous) outcomes: It has two parts:

Part I: What is the average weight of students?

You are interested to know the average weight of students in a class (just a curiosity-driven question – may be used to decide the capacity of lift just outside the class). There are 200 boys and 100 girls in the class. Someone finds out that the average weight of boys is 70 kg, whereas average weight of girls is 40 kg. So, what will be the average weight of the class? Some students will answer 55 kg; others will answer 60 kg. The second answer is trickier (and correct): 60 kg. $(200\times70+40\times100)/300$ or $(2\times70+1\times40)/3$. The boys are double in number, and hence, their average weight is to be counted twice but that of girls only once. An average calculated in this way is called 'weighted average'. Meta-analysis is essentially a calculation of weighted average. One factor on which the weight depends is the number of subjects (patients) in the study. In other words, one factor determining weight is the 'sample size' of the study.

Part II: What is the weight for each of two trials?

Consider a situation when two groups of investigators are asked to carry out a 7-year follow-up study to determine whether daily exercise and weight reduction prevent heart attacks. Seven-year follow-up was the most daunting part of the study.

Study 1 – One group comes up with a brilliant idea to do the study at a school, because school children with thousands of enrollees and some teachers at a school are easy to follow, say, from class V to XII. They recruit 2,000 overweight students (and some teachers) and randomise them into two groups: one intervention group (receives daily exercise and weight-reducing diet) and a control group (without the intervention).

Study 2 by the second group of investigators recruits 1,000 overweight people aged >45 years and randomised them into two groups in a similar fashion. Which study is likely to yield more information? Study 2 is likely to yield more information as there are more persons likely to get heart attack (event of interest) in this, whereas the school subjects in study 1 are very unlikely to get heart attack. (Some teachers might!) Therefore, in a meta-analysis, which study should be given more weight? Study 2 should be given more weight than study 1, even though it has only half the sample size of study 1. The weight does depend not only on sample size but also on the information that a study provides. The information content of a study depends on the number of events in the study. Accordingly, the weight assigned to a study in a meta-analysis with binary outcomes is determined by two factors: (1) sample size and (2) no. of events. In case of two studies with the same number of events in each group (intervention and control), the weight will depend on their sample size, but otherwise, the no. of events is more important than sample size.

You need not know the exact formula used for weighting but enough to know that these two things go into the formula determining weight of each study in a meta-analysis.

Sub-step 6(d): Combining Results on Benefits, Risks and Tolerability

Having decided upon the formula for combining, the results on all important outcomes including beneficial and adverse effects as well as tolerability (if applicable) are combined.

Sub-step 6(e): Subgroup Analyses

One of the advantages of meta-analysis is its power to allow subgroup analysis. It can have data from such large number of patients that the effects may be examined according to subgroups based on the type of patients (children and adults) or interventions (streptokinase and t-PA).

Step 7: Interpretation of the Results

This is similar to the interpretation of a single study, except that a meta-analysis provides an opportunity to examine consistency of the results across studies, across different subgroups of patients, across various outcome categories and in relation to the quality of studies. Some reviewers provide a plot of results with only the best studies included and then with successive inclusion of varying level of quality of the studies.

There is a need to keep in mind that meta-analysis is most often a retrospective study (now prospective meta-analysis is also appearing in literature). The sources of error in any retrospective study are several, and hence, firm conclusions can only be made with P values much less than 0.05, which is the conventional level of statistical significance. Many experts recommend a P value of 0.001 or less for making firm conclusions, but I think it may depend on the costs and risk of the intervention and the available evidence external to the studies included in the meta-analysis.

Advantages of Meta-analysis

The main advantage of meta-analysis is increased power (strength) arising from the combination of results from several studies. The combined result may be more precise and, hence, often conclusive, even when individual studies are inconclusive. There is increased power for overall as well as subgroup analyses. Conclusive results of a meta-analysis on a topic may obviate the need for a new trial and expedite application of the research results. Even when results are inconclusive, meta-analysis defines the area for research, generates hypotheses to be tested and informs the future research regarding limitations of the available evidence. Meta-analysis requires a relook at each included study and a comparison across studies. This may settle or explain controversies.

Experts feel that the results of meta-analysis have greater generalisability because it is based on a variety of study populations. The summary provided by a meta-analysis on a topic is useful for economic evaluation, decision analysis and clinical practice guidelines.

Limitations of Meta-analysis

All meta-analyses have to deal with publication bias, that is, positive results are published more often than the negative ones. Thus, a meta-analysis based on only published trials may yield a false-positive result. Such instances have already occurred in medical literature.

Another limitation is its infeasibility when the studies have used different outcomes or have measured outcomes differently or the reports do not report some vital aspect of the study and authors are unavailable or apathetic.

A problem often called 'combining apples and oranges' refers to combining very dissimilar studies, which may drown a genuine positive result into an overall false-negative conclusion.

References

1. Mason JW, Peters FA. Antiarrhythmic efficacy of encainide in patients with refractory recurrent ventricular tachycardia. Circulation. 1981;63:670–5.
2. Echt DS, Liebson PR, Mitchell LB, et al. Mortality and morbidity in patients receiving encainide, flecainide, or placebo. The Cardiac Arrhythmia Suppression Trial. N Engl J Med. 1991;324:781–8.
3. Prasad K, Shrivastava A. A surgery for primary supratentorial intracerebral haemorrhage (Cochrane review). In: The Cochrane Library, issue 4. Oxford: Update Software; 2000.

Further Reading

Cooper HM, Rosenthal R. Statistical versus traditional procedures for summarizing research findings. Psychol Bull. 1980;87:442–9.

Counsell CE, Clarke MJ, Slattery J, Sandercock PA. The miracle of DICE therapy for acute stroke: fact or fictional product of subgroup analysis? BMJ. 1994;309:1677–81.

Dickersin K. The existence of publication bias and risk factors for its occurrence. JAMA. 1990;263:1385–9.

Egger M, Davey Smith G, Altman DG, editors. Systematic reviews in health care: meta-analysis in context. 2nd ed. London: BMJ Books; 2000.

Guyatt G, Rennie D, editors. User's guides to the medical literature: a manual for evidence-based clinical practice. Chicago: AMA Press; 2002. (www.ama-assn.org).

Irwig L, Tosteson AN, Gatsonis C, et al. Guidelines for meta-analyses evaluating diagnostic tests. Ann Intern Med. 1994;120:667–76.

Oxman AD, Guyatt GH. The science of reviewing research. Ann N Y Acad Sci. 1993;703:125–33; discussion 133–4.

Peto R. Why do we need systematic overviews of randomized trials? Stat Med. 1987;6:233–44.

Further Reading

Chapter 11
Meta-analysis: Critical Appraisal

This chapter deals with the critical appraisal of a meta-analysis of treatment studies that are randomised.

Relevance

When checking the relevance, you ask whether the population, intervention, comparison and outcome of the meta-analysis are matching those of your clinical question or not.

Validity Assessment

The following questions need to be asked and their answers examined while critically appraising a meta-analysis or systematic review:

Q1. Did the review (meta-analysis) address a focused clinical question?
Q2. Was the search for relevant studies comprehensive and well documented?
Q3. Were the included studies of high methodological quality?
Q4. Was there a good agreement between reviewers in selection and assessment of studies?
Q5. Were the combined results combinable (similar from study to study)?

Q.1. Did the Review (Meta-analysis) Address a Focused Clinical Question?

The strength of a meta-analysis comes from the ability to combine the results across studies. However, one has to be cautious not to combine apples and arranges. If the

K. Prasad, *Fundamentals of Evidence-Based Medicine*,
DOI 10.1007/978-81-322-0831-0_11, © Springer India 2013

effect is similar across studies, the results support combining; if not, they raise the questions like combining apples and oranges.

1A. Why do we ask this question?
The question is important from two (the internal and external validity) points of view. First, if the effects are dissimilar across the studies and if the underlying biology suggests that the effects would be dissimilar – yet the reviewers combine the study results to get a summary – then the summary is likely to be misleading (a threat to internal validity). Such a summary would not be applicable to patients.

1. Internal validity here would refer to the extent to which the summary result reflects the 'true' effects across the studies in the meta-analysis.
2. External validity refers to the extent to which the summary results would apply to patients (and/or interventions) outside those in the studies' (Lack of focus in the question may pose a threat to both internal as well as external validity).

1B. How do we answer the question?
In the methods section look for precise statement of what range of patients, interventions and outcomes the reviewer has considered for the meta-analysis, then consider whether it is plausible that the effects across the range of patients, interventions and outcomes could be similar. If the answer is yes, then the review is addressing a focused clinical question, otherwise not.

Here, some caution is necessary in answering the question. No matter how similar are patients, interventions and outcomes, there would still be some differences across the included studies. You should not reject the review without looking at the results. Our knowledge of biology is usually so incomplete that results may differ from our expectation. Also, a narrowly focused review may have the limitations of a subgroup analysis that often yield false-positive conclusions. Therefore, a broadly focused review is preferable to a narrowly focused review. For example, the role of antiplatelet events (aspirin, dipyridamole, etc.) in arterial thrombosis (stroke, myocardial infarction, etc.) may be a reasonable topic for meta-analysis, but effects of chemotherapy on all cancers are not, because chemotherapy is effective for some cancers but not for others.

1C. How do we interpret the answer?
If the question is reasonably focused, you proceed without hesitation. Even if the question appears too broad, it is advisable to proceed further and revisit this question while evaluating similarity of results across the studies.

Q.2. Was the Search for Relevant Studies Comprehensive and Well Documented?

A comprehensive search would require searching for both published and unpublished studies. The search should be documented so that if you (or someone) had doubt about its comprehensives or wanted to replicate the meta-analysis, you could replicate the search and check the yield.

2A. Why do we ask this question?
The question is important to ensure that the review does not suffer from publication bias (positive studies are published more easily than negative ones). There are examples of meta-analyses, which predicted very strong effects that were not observed in a subsequent clinical trial. For example, a meta-analysis predicted that magnesium sulphate would be highly effective in reducing mortality following acute myocardial infarction. A subsequent clinical trial did not find such effects. The meta-analysis has been alleged to have 'publication bias' [1].

2B. How do we answer the question?
Read the methods section to find how the reviewers searched for studies. A good search may include:

(a) Electronic databases, such as MEDLINE, EMBASE and the Cochrane Controlled Trials Register
(b) Textbooks and monographs
(c) Reference lists of retrieved articles
(d) Contact with experts
(e) Abstracts of conferences/meetings
(f) Contact with pharmaceutical companies
(g) Hand searching

Experts and pharmaceutical companies help to provide 'in press' and co-published studies. (There are statistical methods to explore possibility of publication bias, but they are beyond the scope of this book.) Non-English language studies also need to be included in the review.

2C. How do we interpret the answer?
If the search is not comprehensive (e.g. limited only to English language), then findings of the review may be considered only tentative.

Q.3. Were the Included Studies of High Methodological Quality?

Poor design or conduct of the included studies may compromise the validity of the review. The quality is relevant in two of the steps of meta-analysis or SR:

(a) While selecting studies for inclusion into the review
(b) While assessing the quality of the included studies

3A. How do we answer the question?
Read the methods section of the review to find whether reviewers used a certain selection criteria for including only good-quality studies. Usually, a study design is used as selection criteria, e.g. randomised controlled trials.

Reviewers should also assess whether the studies have been conducted properly. Thus, even for randomised trials, quality needs to be critically appraised using the criteria and questions given in the therapy section of this book.

3B. How do we interpret the answer?
If methodological quality was not assessed, you should doubt the results of the meta-analysis. If this was done, you may like to see if there was good agreement between two reviewers. A kappa of around 0.6 or more would be acceptable. The next thing is to see whether the reviewers have used the quality score in excluding, or weighting or prioritising the studies while combining them.

Q.4. Was There a Good Agreement Between Reviewers in Selection and Assessment of Studies?

At least two reviewers should independently select and assess the studies for the review. This is done to avoid bias in selection of the studies and assessment of their quality. Two reviewers should also do the data extraction from the included studies. There should be high agreement between the reviewers in all these activities. Some agreement would occur by chance alone, and therefore, they should present some measure of agreement beyond chance (Kappa or phi). Kappa and phi above 0.6 are considered adequate. You should look for report of one or both of the measures in the results section of the review.

Kappa and phi are 'measures of chance-corrected agreement'. This concept may be new for you, but just remember that the value of Kappa and phi range from −1 (extreme disagreement) to +1 (prefect agreement). Values between 0.6 and 0.8 are considered substantial, above 0.8, almost perfect. Details are beyond the scope of this book.

Q.5. Were the Combined Results Combinable (Similar from Study to Study)?

Reviewers should not combine apples and oranges. In other words, if results are very different from study to study, it is important to know why they are different, rather than the average of all.

5A. Why do we ask this question?
The goal of a meta-analysis is too often to provide a single best estimate of the effect of a treatment that clinicians can rely on to make clinical decisions. The estimate usually comes from taking a weighted average of the effects across the studies. Taking average makes sense only if the effects are more or less similar across the studies. If the effects are very different, the average may be meaningless or misleading. For example, if thrombolytic therapy in ischaemic stroke was found harmful in some studies, and helpful in other studies, the average may show equivocal results, which may actually be misleading. There has indeed been a debate on whether studies of streptokinase (three trials stopped prematurely due to excess deaths in the streptokinase group) and t-PA (studies showing some benefit) in acute ischaemic stroke should

be combined. Many reviewers would object to combining them. Therefore, the question whether the results are similar from study to study must be examined.

This should not be interpreted as all studies showing clear benefit or all showing clear harm. [If such is a case, the conclusion may seem obvious, even without a meta-analysis]. The idea is that they should not be disparate or widely different. They may well be a mixture of inconclusive and benefit-showing studies. In any case, similarities and differences among the studies should always be examined. This is what is called the issue of combinability or similarity.

5B. How do we answer the question?

To answer the question about similarity, you can use four methods. They are complementary to each other. They are as follows:

(i) Examine study design, study population, intervention, outcomes and study methodology:
Effects may differ depending on study designs because the degree of bias in the data differs from one design to another. Randomised controlled studies are generally less susceptible to bias than the case–control studies. Similarly effects may vary due to differences in study population, type and dose of interventions and types of outcome measures and timing of their measurement. For example, patient with acute ischaemic stroke may have differences in results depending on whether they receive t-PA within 3 or 3–6 h after onset, whether they receive a dose of 0.9 mg/kg body weight or 1.1 mg/kg, whether you measure death as outcome or disability free survival and whether outcome is measured at 3 or 6 months after randomisation. Also, whether the outcome measurement is blinded or open and whether randomisation was concealed or unconcealed may make a difference in the results.

(ii) Examine the point estimates in the forest plot: If they are close to each other, the results are likely to be similar.

(iii) Examine whether the confidence intervals (usually 95 %) overlap: If you can draw a line or a pair of lines through the confidence intervals of the various studies so that it or they pass through or touch all of them means that the confidence intervals overlap. It tells you that the data is consistent with one (or a range of) result common to all studies. This indicates that the results across the studies may be similar.

(iv) Test of homogeneity or heterogeneity: The above methods are based on clinical or common sense. There is also a formal statistical test called test of homogeneity (simpler term would have been test of similarity). This test asks the questions: Are the differences likely due to chance? The answer comes in the form of *P* value. If the *P* value is more than 0.05 or 0.10, the differences may be considered likely to be due to chance, and study results are considered combinable.
You should note that the results of the test may sometimes be misleading. If the number of and size of studies are small, the test may not pick up even important differences. On the other hand, if the number and size of studies are large, the test may overly highlight even the small differences. However, the former situation is more common than the latter.

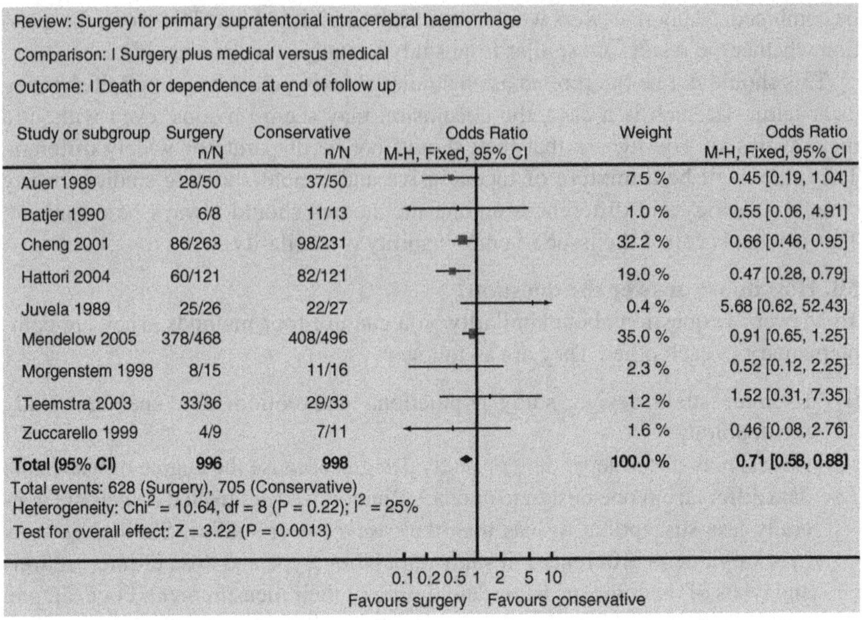

Fig. 11.1 Forest plot of a meta-analysis

(v) Another statistic, perhaps more reasonable than the test of homogeneity, is I^2. This indicates the percentage of variability in effect estimates that is due to underlying differences in effect rather than chance [2]. The following is a rough guide for the interpretation if I^2:

0 % to 40 %: probably not important.
30 % to 60 %: moderate heterogeneity.
50 % to 90 %: substantial heterogeneity.
75 % to 100 %: considerable heterogeneity.

The above ranges are overlapping, because importance of the observed value of I square depends on magnitude and direction of effects and strength of evidence of heterogeneity, such as *P* value of chi-squared test.

However, even I square may sometimes give misleading results. Hence, visual inspection of point estimates and confidence intervals is very important. For example, denoted as square in Fig. 11.1, you see that the point estimates are close to each other, confidence intervals are overlapping and test of heterogeneity ($P=0.22$) and I^2 of 25 % all suggest no serious concern about heterogeneity.

At the end (in Cochrane reviews, last line of first few columns), the forest plots present total number of events and patients, results of test of heterogeneity, as *P* values, I^2 and *P* value associated with the summary estimate. The interpretation of I^2 has been presented above. There are two *P* values, sometimes leading to confusion in their interpretation. One *P* value refers to test of homogeneity where the null hypothesis is that 'there is no difference in effects across the studies'. You do not wish to reject this hypothesis, because if you reject this, there will be serious concern about the justification of summarising the results. P value <0.05 would suggest rejection, and hence, you want $P>0.05$ or better still >0.10. The second P value (lower one in Cochrane review) refers to the overall results. There is the null hypothesis is 'there is no difference in results between the two interventions'. Most of the time, you wish to reject this hypothesis and conclude that the new (experimental) intervention does make a difference. Therefore, here you wish to see P value <0.05.

The above discussion will help you to understand a forest plot.

5C. How do you interpret the answers?

If all methods suggest that the study results are similar, then you believe the summary. If the test of homogeneity suggests dissimilarity, then don't believe the results unless you are convinced that point estimates are close to each other and confidence intervals overlap and there is no explanation available for the dissimilarity.

When all methods suggest dissimilarity, the authors of the meta-analysis should provide explanations for the observed differences. Again the explanations may be due to differences in population, intervention, outcome, study design or methodology. The search for explanation may sometimes be misleading (details are beyond the scope of this book). In any case, you should not believe the overall summary estimate for very dissimilar effects across studies. More studies are required to clarify the situation.

Assessment of Results, Applicability and Application (What Is the Information and How Can You Apply the Results to Patient Care?)

The main learning point here is to learn interpretation of a forest plot (also called 'blobbogram'). In a typical forest plot of a meta-analysis, you will find five or six columns:

1. The first column lists the studies usually identified with their first author's name and year of publication. The studies may sometimes be grouped into two or more subgroups based on a characteristic of patients or interventions.
2. The second column gives the number of patients with outcome/total number in the intervention group. Usually experimental intervention is presented in the second column.
3. The third column is similar to the second but the placebo or control group data are presented.
4. The fourth column presents results of individual studies using an effect measure (either a difference measure or a ratio measure). There is a vertical 'line of no effect' (also called 'null effect line'). Results on one side of the line (usually left) favour the experimental intervention, while the opposite side (usually the right) favours the control intervention or placebo.
   Results from each study have a point (in Cochrane reviews, the form is square and size of the square is proportion to the weight of the study in determining the study estimate) and a line extending on either side of the line. You would know from our

discussion – Chap. 4 – that the point is the observed effect in the study and is called 'point estimate' and the lines represent the confidence interval (usually 95 %). At the bottom of this column, you will find a summary estimate with its point estimate and confidence interval (CI). In Cochrane review, the summary estimate is indicated in the form of a diamond with its centre representing the point estimate and ends representing the confidence limits (i.e. ends of CI usually 95 %).

5. There is one column indicating the weight of the study in determining the summary estimate. Usually this is the fifth column placed usually right to results but may sometimes be placed on their left.
6. The last column gives the numerical value of the point estimates and CI for each study and also the summary estimate.

The rest of issues and interpretation here are similar to those you used for a single randomised study of therapy (refer to Chap. 6).

References

1. Egger M, Davey Smith G, Schneider M, Minder C. Bias in meta-analysis detected by a simple, graphical test. BMJ. 1997;315:629–34.
2. Higgins JP, Thompson SG, Deeks JJ, Altman DG. Measuring of inconsistency in meta-analyses. BMJ. 2003;327:557–60.

Further Reading

Detsky AS, Naylor CD, O'Rourke K, McGeer AJ, L'Abbe KA. Incorporating variations in the quality of individual randomized trials into meta-analysis. J Clin Epidemiol. 1992;45:255–65.

Dickersin K. How important is publication bias? A synthesis of available data. AIDS Educ Prev. 1997;9 suppl 1:15–21.

Guyatt G, Rennie D, editors. User's guides to the medical literature: a manual for evidence-based clinical practice. Chicago: AMA Press; 2002. (www.ama-assn.org).

Juni P, Witschi A, Bloch R, Egger M. The hazards of scoring the quality of clinical trials for meta-analysis. JAMA. 1999;282:1054–60.

Kunz R, Oxman AD. The unpredictability paradox: review of empirical comparisons of randomised and non-randomised clinical trials. BMJ. 1998;317:1185–90.

Moher D, Jadad AR, Nichol G, Penman M, Tugwell P, Walsh S. Assessing the quality of randomized controlled trials: an annotated bibliography of scales and checklists. Control Clin Trials. 1995;16:62–73.

Moher D, Pham B, Jones A, et al. Does quality of reports of randomised trials affect estimates of intervention efficacy reported in meta-analyses? Lancet. 1998;352:609–13.

Oxman AD, Guyatt GH. A consumer's guide to subgroup analyses. Ann Intern Med. 1992;116:78–84.

Stern JM, Simes RJ. Publication bias: evidence of delayed publication in a cohort study of clinical research projects. BMJ. 1997;315:640–5.

Yusuf S, Wittes J, Probstfield J, Tyroler HA. Analysis and interpretation of treatment effects in subgroups of patients in randomized clinical trials. JAMA. 1991;266:93–8.

Chapter 12
Prognosis

Introduction

Knowledge of prognosis helps in:

1. Care of individual patients:
   (a) For counselling patients (and/or their relatives) about their likely fate
   (b) Guiding our diagnostic and treatment decisions (e.g. withholding invasive tests or toxic treatments from those destined to have good prognosis without any treatments)
2. Comparing outcomes in certain groups of patients (treated in one hospital vs. another) to assess the quality of care

This section focuses on how to critically appraise articles that contain prognostic information that will be useful in counselling patients.

Validity Assessment

Q.1. Was There Any Selection Bias (Or Is the Study Sample Biased)?

Selection bias occurs when the patients under study are systematically different from the underlying population. This does not necessarily mean a conscious attempt on the part of the researchers to select a biased sample. Most often it occurs subconsciously because of the way study sample is assembled. Patients are included in a study because they both have a disease and are currently available (possibly because they are attending a clinic or a hospital).

K. Prasad, *Fundamentals of Evidence-Based Medicine*,
DOI 10.1007/978-81-322-0831-0_12,

1A. Why do we ask the question?
If the study sample is biased, then the results will be systematically different from what would have happened with unbiased sample. A disease begins in a member of a population. Let us call this a base population. The patients in a study include only those who are available for study some time after their disease began. For fatal conditions, such patients are the ones who are fortunate enough to have survived, and for diseases that remit, the patients are the ones who are unfortunate enough to have persistent disease. So, the biased sample may consist of only patients who survive and in whom the disease survives. This is why a term 'survivor bias' is sometimes used to describe this bias. Survivor bias may be a threat to validity of the conclusions of the study.

1B. How do we answer the question?
To detect selection bias in prognosis studies, look to see how the patients were assembled and what selection criteria were used. You ask: Is the criteria such that some patients from the base population would be missed because they recovered or died? If selection criteria are vague, the risk of biased sample is high. If it is clear, you consider the extent to which it will miss the serious or mild cases. For example, a hospital-based study of prognosis after stroke may have the criteria to include patients within the first month of onset. The patients who come in the third or fourth week after onset are those who survived the first 2 weeks and also did not recover. Many patients who developed stroke in the base population during the same week as these patients are not represented in the study. However, if the criteria include only those patients presenting within 72 h after onset may not suffer from the survivor bias to the same extent as above study. You should consider these aspects and decide whether there is high or low likelihood of bias in the sample selection.

1C. How do we interpret the answer?
If the likelihood of bias is high, then the results of the study are not useful to counsel the patients. However, there is perhaps no prognostic study, completely free from selection bias, and hence, you should be willing to accept a study with low likelihood of bias and assess further with the questions below.

Q.2. Did the Researchers Consider All Important Prognostic Factors?

Prognosis of most diseases is multifactorial. There are many prognostic factors that need to be considered while determining prognosis in an individual patient.

2A. Why do we ask the question?
If researchers did not consider certain important prognostic factors, the outcome rate of the study and prognostic prediction on its basis may not be valid. For example, if a study of brain haemorrhage reports 50 % mortality, but half of the patients

are fully conscious and they all survive, whereas the other half are all comatose and they all die, the 50 % mortality rate may be valid for the group as a whole but not valid for a fully conscious patient or a comatose patient.

Researchers may consider the various prognostic factors in one of the two ways:

(a) If there are few (one to three) important factors, they may form subgroups of patients according to the factors and provide outcome rates for each subgroup (referred to as risk stratification).
(b) If there are many prognostic factors, use multivariable (regression) analysis to determine the most powerful predictors.

2B. How do we answer the question?
Based on your knowledge and experience of the condition, can you think of important prognostic factors that the researchers have ignored? If the answer is yes, the results may not be valid for applying to individual patients. Also look for results presented either as subgroups (or use of one of the multivariable analyses). Subgroup outcome rates may help you to get closer to your patient's prognosis.

2C. How do we interpret the answer?
First of all, keep in mind that most of the time there is no way to be 100 % correct in predicting your individual patient's prognosis. However, if outcome rates of subgroups are given, decide which subgroup your patient belongs to and use the outcome rate of that subgroup in communicating with your patient or his relatives. (Multivariable analysis is beyond the scope of this book.)

Q.3. Were Losses to Follow-Up Sufficiently Small?

Follow-up is a key factor in the validity and usefulness of a prognosis paper. There are two aspects of follow-up that need attention:

(i) The losses to follow-up: The number of patients lost to follow-up threatens validity of the study.
(ii) Length of follow-up: Too short a follow-up may compromise the usefulness of the study. (Length of follow-up is discussed in the applicability section.)

Here we discuss the number lost to follow-up:

3A. Why do we ask this question?
If too many patients are lost to follow-up, the validity of the study may be threatened. This is so because the patients lost to follow-up tend to be systematically different from those who turn up for follow-up. Patients do not turn up for follow-up because they die, because they recover fully or because they are dissatisfied with the care and go to some other doctor or hospital. The larger the number of patients lost to follow-up relative to the number who suffered an adverse event, the greater is the threat to the study's validity.

3B. How do we answer the question?
Look at the results section. Researchers describe (they should) how many patients they started with and how many were lost to follow-up. Sometimes, they do not mention anything about the lost to follow-up. Usually such studies have significant number of patients lost to follow-up. Validity of such studies remains open to question.

3C. How do we interpret the answer?
Some losses to follow-up are very common. The question is how many is too many? To answer this question, do a sensitivity analysis. Assume that all those lost to follow-up had the adverse outcome (bad prognosis), what would be the rate with bad prognosis, and then assume all had the favourable outcome (good prognosis), then what would be the rate? The true rate lies between the two rates. If the clinical implications (your response, patients' choice) remain the same with either rate, then the losses to follow-up do not threaten the validity of the conclusion. If the clinical implications are different with the two rates, then the number lost to follow-up were too many.

Q.4. Was the Measurement of Outcome(s) Reliable and Valid (Unbiased)?

Bias may occur in the measurement of outcome if the criteria for defining the outcome are subjective and the assessor is aware of the presence of certain prognostic factors. Certain outcomes like death are not subject to bias, while others like disability or quality of life are more likely to be so.

4A. Why do we ask this question?
Obviously, if the outcome measurement is biased, the rate of outcome event would be either an underestimate or overestimate. It won't be the true rate.

4B. How do we answer the question?
Look for two things: (a) the criteria for measuring the outcome and (b) whether the assessors of outcome were blinded to the presence or absence of baseline prognostic factors. Some outcomes like death are clear-cut, but some like transient ischaemic attack or angina pectoris require some judgment. Ideally, reliability (e.g. interobserver and intraobserver agreement) and validity of these judgments should have been established prior to starting the prognostic study. If scales are used to determine the outcome, their reliability and validity should be reported in the study.

Blinding to the baseline prognostic factors is desirable, but some such factors can be difficult to blind. For example, age and sex of the patient would be obvious to the assessors even on telephone. However, wherever possible, to avoid bias in the measurement of subjective outcomes, the study should report the attempts made by the researchers.

4C. How to interpret the answer?
If outcome measures are objective (like death), you may accept that there is no likelihood of bias. The more subjective are the outcomes, the more is the likelihood of bias.

Results Assessment

Q.1. What Is (Are) the Probability(–ies) of the Outcomes?

It would be fantastic to be able to summarise the prognosis of a disease as a single number, usually rate[1]: the percent of people experiencing an outcome event. The rates commonly used to describe prognosis are as follows:

(a) Five-year survival: Percent of patients surviving 5 years from some defined time point in the course of their disease.
(b) Case fatality: Percent of patients with a disease who dies of it. Those patients who die of unrelated cause are not included in this.
(c) All cause mortality: Percent of patients in a cohort who die of any cause.
(d) Response: Percent of patients showing some evidence of improvement following an intervention.
(e) Remission: Percent of patients becoming free of any evidence of the activity of a disease.
(f) Recurrence: Percent of patients who have return of disease activity after a period of remission.

These rates are sometimes referred to as summary rates, because they summarise the experience of a groups of patients in one number.

If all (or nearly all) the events occur within a short length of follow-up, e.g. in hours or days or weeks, then the summary rates are acceptable and meaningful measures of prognosis. The good point about these rates is their simplicity; you can memorise them easily and communicate succinctly. The downside of these rates is that large differences in prognosis can be hidden within similar summary rates. For example, Fig. 12.1 shows 5-year survival for patients with dissecting aneurysm and AIDS.

For each condition, about 10 % of the patients are alive at 5 years, but the survival pattern is considerably different. For dissecting aneurysm, early mortality is very high, but if they survive the first few months, their risk of dying levels up (becomes constant). On the other hand, patients with AIDS die throughout the 5 years. The fact of death at 5 years gives the same percentage; but the time-to-death (survival) has been different for the two conditions.

To overcome this drawback, time-to-death (=survival) is analysed for a cohort of patients and is presented in the form of a graph, called 'survival curve'. The form of analysis that yields the curve is called survival analysis. Survival curves are usually the probability of surviving (without the event 'death') on the vertical axis (but sometimes the proportion with, rather than without, the outcome event is indicated on the vertical axis). In either case, the horizontal axis has the period of time since the beginning of observation.

[1]Strictly speaking, these are not rates, but proportions. However, in common usage, often the words recurrence rate, remission rate, etc., are used.

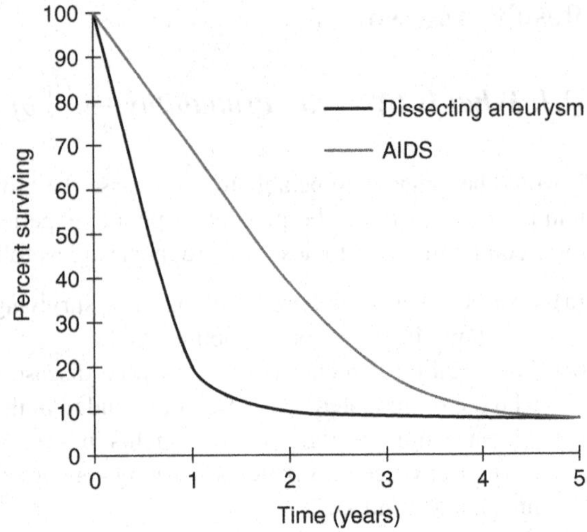

Fig. 12.1 Of two conditions with the same 5-year survival rate of 10 %

The details of how the survival curves are formed are beyond the scope of this book, but certain points to be kept in mind when interpreting survival curves are as follows:

(i) The vertical axis does not represent the actual percent surviving for an actual cohort, but the estimated probability of surviving for members of a hypothetical cohort.
(ii) Often, the number of patients at risk at various points in time is shown below the horizontal axis. The estimates on the left-hand side of curve are sound, because more patients are at risk during this time. But at the tail of the curve, on the right, the number of patients on whom the estimation is based is often small because fewer patients are available for follow-up for that length of time. As a result, estimates of survival towards the end of the follow-up period are less precise than in the earlier period.
(iii) The survival analysis methodology can be used to analyse not only time-to-death (=survival) but also time-to-any event, and the results can be presented as a 'survival curve'. The events may be remission, recurrence, stroke or acute myocardial infarction.
(iv) Survival curve can be used to describe survival after any length of time – 1, 2, 3 or 5 years. This gives a more complete and detailed description of prognosis.
(v) When percent (probability) of having an event, rather than not having it, is presented, the curve starts at 'zero' and sweeps upward and to the right.

Q.2. What Is the Margin of Error?

The margin of error in the determination (or estimation) of rates is given by 95 % confidence intervals (CIs). The interpretation of CIs can be done using the methods described in Chap. 4.

The 95 % CIs around the points on the survival curve are (and should be) presented at various points on the survival curve. As discussed above, the intervals will be narrower (more precise) on the left side of the curve than on the right side, towards the tail.

Applicability Assessment (Can You Apply the Results to Patient Care?)

Q.1. Were the Study Patients and Their Management Similar to Those in Your Practice?

The results are applicable if the patient and treatment characteristics in your setting are similar to the ones in the study. You should judge this by examining the description of the patients and their management in the study. If the description is inadequate or the characteristics differ from your own patients and settings, then the applicability of the results is questionable.

Q.2. Was Follow-Up Sufficiently Long?

Follow-up must be long enough for all or nearly all clinically relevant events to occur; otherwise the reported rate will underestimate the true one. Of course, if death is an outcome, one cannot follow up patients till all of them die; but a reasonably long follow-up is necessary for the results to be useful. Even if a study passes the validity criteria, but the length of follow-up is very short, the study results may not be useful, because you and your patients may be interested in prognosis over a long period of time.

Q.3. How Can You Use the Results in the Management of Your Patients?

Knowledge of prognosis helps in three ways in caring for your patients:

(i) If the patient's prognosis without treatment is excellent, you may decide not to treat the patient. For example, asymptomatic colonic diverticula have such a good prognosis that you may not treat them.
(ii) If the patient's prognosis is uniformly poor (e.g. patients with massive brain haemorrhage with sign of brain death), you may decide to start discussing with the family about organ donations, disconnecting from ventilator, etc.
(iii) For patients' with intermediate prognosis, you may use the prognostic prediction to weigh the risks versus benefits of a treatment. In doing so, keep

in mind that the rates from any prognosis study is derived from a group of patients, some of whom had the poor outcome and some had good outcome. The rate is an average over all the patients. There is always a question to consider: To what extent does this average rate apply to your patient? The more your patient is like the average patient in the study or one of its described subgroup, the more is the applicability of the rate from the relevant patient group of the study. The extent to which your patient differs from the described group or subgroup of study patients determines the extent to which you need to upscale or downscale the reported rate to counsel your patients.

Application

If your patient is similar to the average patient in the study, you can quote the overall results of the study as your patient's prognosis. If your patient is not like the average patient of the study, you have two options: either use the equation derived from the study (if authors report this) with the variables of your patient or use your clinical judgment to upscale or downscale the rate reported in the study according to your patient's prognostic factors.

Further Reading

Concato J, Feinstein AR, Holford TR. The risk of determining risk with multivariable models. Ann Intern Med. 1993;118:201–10.

Ellenberg JH, Nelson KB. Sample selection and the natural history of disease: studies of febrile seizures. JAMA. 1980;243:1337–40.

Guyatt G, Rennie D, editors. User's guides to the medical literature: a manual for evidence-based clinical practice. Chicago: AMA Press; 2002. (www.ama-assn.org).

Guyatt GH, Feeny DH, Patrick DL. Measuring health-related quality of life. Ann Intern Med. 1993;118:622–9.

Kopecky SL. The natural history of lone atrial fibrillation: a population-based study over three decades. N Engl J Med. 1987;317:669–74.

Kriel RL, Krach LE, Jones-Saete C. Outcome of children with prolonged unconsciousness and vegetative states. Pediatr Neurol. 1993;9:362–8.

Laupacis A, Wells G, Richardson S, Tugwell P. Users' guides to the medical literature. V. How to use an article about prognosis. JAMA. 1994;272:234–7.

Meador CK. The art and science of nondisease. N Engl J Med. 1965;272:92.

Walsh JS, Welch G, Larson EB. Survival of outpatients with Alzheimer-type dementia. Ann Intern Med. 1990;113:429–34.

Wolmark N, et al. The prognostic significance of preoperative carcinoembryonic antigen levels in colorectal cancer. Results from the NSABP clinical trials. Ann Surg. 1984;199:375–82.

Chapter 13
Advanced Topics

Fixed and Random Effects Models

Let us begin with a story. Some years ago, banks came up with a new concept for fixed deposits. The concept was to give interest on interest. This was called 'compound interest'. Before this concept, the interest was calculated only on the principal – and the approach was called 'simple interest'. One may call them 'simple interest model' and 'compound interest model'. As you can see, these are two different concepts underlying the computation of the maturity amount. In the simple interest model, there is only one source of interest, i.e. the principal, whereas in the compound interest model, there are two sources of interest: the principal as well as the interest earned periodically.

Computation is based on different formulae such that the formula for simple interest uses only the principal as the source of interest and in the compound interest model, there are two sources of interest – first, the principal and, second, the interest earned over certain fixed periods (say, every 3 months).

The practical difference between the two is that the maturity amount is more in the compound interest than in the simple interest. Thus, you can see that the differences between simple interest model and compound interest model are conceptual, computational and practical. Similarly, the differences between fixed and random effects models may be described as:

- Conceptual
- Computational
- Practical

Conceptually, in the fixed effects model, the studies are believed to estimate the same underlying true effect, and all the differences in the effect estimates are due only to differences in the sample size. In random effects model, the studies estimate an effect that in itself is assumed to be a random variable with a certain distribution. Alternatively, in random effects model, the studies conceptually represent a sample of a large (infinite) number of possible studies on the questions, whereas in fixed

K. Prasad, *Fundamentals of Evidence-Based Medicine*,
DOI 10.1007/978-81-322-0831-0_13, © Springer India 2013

effects model, the studies at hand represent the total number of studies on the question. Put another way, we consider the sample as the only reason for differences in results among the studies, whereas in random effects model, we consider a sample as one reason for differences but also consider that there are other reasons for the differences that are not known.

Computationally, in fixed effects model, only one source of differences in the effect measure is considered, that is, the sample size, whereas in the random effects model, two sources of differences are considered, viz. the sample size and the variation of the effects between the studies.

Practically, the random effects model yields a wider confidence interval than the fixed effects model, and the point estimate may be only slightly different. Moreover, in the fixed effects model, the small studies get relatively more weight than in random effects model. Some experts argue for using mixed models, in which known reasons for differences in effects are considered and treated as 'fixed', and in addition consideration is given to some reasons as yet unknown, for the differences. I have not seen any meta-analysis in medicine using the mixed model, and commonly used software does not have this feature.

You may ask: Which model is better to use? Each model has its supporters. Some experts favour the use of 'fixed effects' model, while others favour the use of 'random effects model'. When there is little or no difference in results across the included studies, both models yield the same results. However, when there are important differences, random effects model is more conservative than fixed effects. Certainly, when there is heterogeneity across study results, and a decision is made to perform meta-analysis, then random effects model should be used. Whenever in doubt, I recommend using both and accept the results if both models yield the same finding. If findings differ between the models, it is better to wait for some more studies before concluding anything.

Hypothesis Testing

Let us begin with an analogy. In a diagnostic test, you use a gold standard. What is the function of a gold standard test? The gold standard tells you the 'true' state, i.e. whether the patient actually has the disease or doesn't have it. Once you know the truth, you can determine as to whether a positive test result is 'true positive' or 'false positive' and similarly whether a negative tests result is true negative or false negative. However, in some situations, it is impossible to exactly know the truth; however, the truth does exist. We conduct studies to discover this truth. You can visualise the study as a diagnostic test, being done to diagnose (discover) the truth. The study will give you some result – it may be positive or negative. The positive result may be true positive or false positive. Likewise, the negative result may be true negative or false negative. (The difference between a diagostic test and a study is that the gold standard test results can be known – i.e. truth can be ascertained or captured.) But when a study tries to capture the truth, we can only plan the study in a way that the risk of false positive and false negative is kept under certain limits. The 2×2 table may be look like this:

		Truth	
		Treatment works (makes a difference)	Treatment does not work (does not make a difference)
Study shows	Treatment works (makes a difference)	True +ve a	False +ve b
	Treatment does not work (does not make a difference)	False −ve c	True −ve d

As you can see, when you plan a study, you must consider two situations when you may land up in error with your study results. One is false-positive error (cell b of the Table). And the second is a false-negative error (cell c of the Table). The false positive error is called type I error, and the false-negative error is called type II error. What can save you from these errors? A large enough sample size. So, while planning your study, you have to calculate sample size based on how much risk of false-positive or false-negative error you would like to take. The risk of false-positive error you take while planning the study is called alpha, and similarly the risk of false-negative error you take is called beta. So, if you want to know what sample size you require for your study, a question will be asked to you: What is the risk of false-positive and false-negative error you are willing to take? In other words, what is your alpha and beta? You might think that you would like them to be zero, but in that case the sample size would be infinity! Then, you might like to know what other researchers do? Well, almost universally, researchers set alpha to be 5 %. What about beta? Usually researchers set them at 10 or 20 %. If you want beta to be 10 %, the sample size will be more than it would be with 20 %. Many students, at first instance, intend to keep beta also at 5 %: But its implication is such a large sample size that is often infeasible and unmanageable. Therefore, single-centre investigator-initiated studies keep beta at 20 %, whereas multicentric sponsored studies often keep it at 10 % or even 5 %. One more small wrinkle? If a diagnostic test has a false-negative error rate of 10 %, what it its sensitivity? You must have figured out 90 %. What is the sensitivity of a diagnostic test if false-negative rate is 20 % – obviously 80 %. Thus, the two are complementary to each other. The notion applies to a study as well. If you want your study to have such a sample size that it is able to detect the truth 90 % of the time, well it will be more sensitive than when you plan to detect it 80 % of the time. When beta is 10 %, sensitivity of the study, i.e. ability to detect the truth, is more than when beta is 20 %. Accordingly, it is quite appropriate that the more the sample size, the more is the sensitivity of the study. The term 'sensitivity' is not used in this context – instead, the term used for this purpose is 'power'. So, power of a study is complementary to beta. When beta = 10 %, power is 90 %; when beta = 20 %, power is 80 %. Typically, researchers plan a study sample with alpha = 5 % and power of 80 or 90 %.

Then let us summarise what you learnt so far:

1. Every study caries some risk of false-positive and false-negative error.
2. False-positive error is called type I error, and false-negative error is called type II error.
3. Risk of false-positive error, which you take or set while calculating a sample size during planning stage of the study, is called alpha.
4. Risk of false-negative error, which you similarly set during planning, is called beta.
5. Power of a study is complement to beta, and it is the ability to detect a difference between two treatment groups when in truth it exists. This is a concept similar to the sensitivity of a diagnostic test.
6. Typically, researchers plan a study with a sample size with alpha = 5 % and power of 80 or 90 %.

Other concepts in planning sample size:

One concept related to this is what is your hypothesis? Suppose you have a hypothesis about IQ of males and females. Your hypothesis may be any of the following:

1. There is no difference in IQ between males and females.
2. There is a difference in IQ between males and females.
3. IQ of males is more than that of females.
4. IQ of females is more than that of males.
5. IQ of females is not less than that of males.

Hypothesis 1 is called 'null hypothesis', which is almost always the basis on which a statistical test is done. No matter what is your hypothesis of interest, statisticians start testing on the basis of an assumption of 'no difference', that is null hypothesis. Thus, null hypothesis is not what you start with. If you do have a hypothesis of no difference, you need to state it like this – IQ of females is equal to that of males or vice versa. This is called 'equivalence' hypothesis. Hypotheses 2, 3 and 4 are 'superiority hypotheses' as they assume that one gender has greater IQ than the other. Hypothesis 5 is termed 'non-inferiority hypothesis', as it only assumes 'not less' IQ for one gender, in this case, females. We will focus our discussion mainly on superiority hypothesis.

In hypothesis 2, if you are saying IQ (males) is not equal to IQ (females), you are happy with difference in either direction: following males or females, both are of interest to you. In hypothesis 3, 4 or 5, you have specified one direction in which your interest lies. In hypothesis 3, you are not bothered to know whether IQ of males is equal or less than that of females. Similarly in hypothesis 4, you specify the direction in favour of females. Accordingly, the statistical tests of your hypothesis will be either two tailed or one tailed. Whenever your hypothesis is not in one direction (non-directional), that means you are interested in either of the two results; the test to be used will be two-tailed. When your hypothesis is in one direction (directional), the test will be one-tailed.

(Don't worry about the origin of the words with 'tail' – suffice it to say that it has nothing to do with animal's tails). Thus, one question you have to answer during the sample size calculation is whether you will use two-tailed or one-tailed test. As you can see, for hypotheses 3, 4 and 5, you will chose one-tailed test, whereas for hypotheses 1 and 2, you will chose two-tailed test. One-tailed test will require smaller sample size than two-tailed test. You may be tempted to chose one-tailed test, but be careful. Many journals do not like this. You will be asked to justify as to why you are interested in only one direction. What do most researchers do? They use two-tailed test.

To summarise, hypothesis testing involves the use of terms alpha, beta, power, superiority/equivalence/non-inferiority and one tailed/two tailed, which we covered in this chapter. Sample size calculation also involves specifying certain figures about patients' (subjects') outcomes (endpoints), which are not covered in this chapter.

Chapter 14
Examples of Critical Appraisal

Clinical Scenario

A 55-year-old man presents to the emergency department with history of chest pain of 4-h duration. You are called to see the patient in the emergency room.

The patient was diagnosed to have hypertension (on routine examinations) 5 years ago. On evaluation (then and subsequently), he has been found to be free of other risk factors for atherosclerotic vascular disease. He was advised salt restriction and ramipril 5 mg OD, with which his BP recorded periodically has been around 135/85 mmHg. He has been well except occasional burning epigastrium, which responds to antacids.

Today in the evening after returning from work, he complained of vague pain over the left side of chest. He initially attributed this to hyperacidity and took two Tsfs. of antacid gel. The pain did not respond, rather it slightly increased over the last 1 h, and he decided to come to the emergency.

On direct questioning, there is no radiation of the pain to the left arm and no associated sweating, vomiting or palpitation. The pain has a burning quality, but he also feels a sense of heaviness over the left parasternal region.

On examination, his pulse rate is 80/min and regular, BP 145/90 mmHg, RR 20/min. and afebrile. Systemic examination is normal. 12-lead ECG is also normal. You admit him to your chest pain assessment unit. You order continuous 12-lead ECG ST segment monitoring and serial measurements of CK-MB mass.

Patient's wife asks: 'What is wrong with him, doctor? Has he got "heart attack"?' You told her that the probability of 'heart attack' is low, but you want to observe him for 6 h before deciding whether to admit him to the hospital or send him home.

You wondered whether you can rule out acute MI after 6 h. You conducted a MEDLINE search and found a recent article: 'Is it possible to exclude a diagnosis of myocardial damage within 6 h of admission to an emergency department?' Diagnostic cohort study by Herren et al. You decided to read this paper.

K. Prasad, *Fundamentals of Evidence-Based Medicine*,
DOI 10.1007/978-81-322-0831-0_14,

Example of Answers to Critical Appraisal of a Diagnosis Paper

Reference: Herren KR, Mackway-Jones K, Richards CR, et al. Is it possible to exclude a diagnosis of myocardial damage within six hours of admission to an emergency department? Diagnostic cohort study. BMJ. 2001;323(7309):372.

Guide	Comments
Are the results of the study valid?	
Did the clinicians face diagnostic uncertainty?	Yes, the physicians at the chest pain assessment unit were uncertain about having ruled out MI. They wanted to know whether it is safe to discharge after a 6-h rule out protocol
Was there blind comparison with an independent gold standard?	*About the 'gold standard'*: Yes, the gold standard for comparison was troponin T test at 48 h. One can ask whether this is an acceptable gold standard. Does it diagnose the condition(s) of concern with sufficient (ideally 100 %) accuracy? What is the condition of concern? In the emergency room, one is concerned about controlling pain and not missing a cardiac condition, which results in cardiac failure or cardiac arrhythmia. Some might argue that the authors should have taken clinically relevant cardiac arrhythmia/failure or sudden cardiac death as the gold standard. Others might consider it adequate because negative troponin test at 48 h. is widely accepted to rule out acute MI which is the major concern in emergency admission
	About the 'blind comparison': We don't know. Authors do not mention whether the laboratory personnel reporting troponin T concentration were unaware of the protocol test results and of the patients' admission/discharge status
Did the results of the test being evaluated influence the decision to perform the gold standard?	No, the decision to perform the gold standard was independent of the protocol test results. But 76 patients could not be subjected to the 'gold standard test'. Authors could trace 61 of these patients 4 weeks or more after discharge. All were apparently free of MI, suggesting that the negative protocol test result was correct. To assure the readers that these patients were not systematically different (more prone to MI) from the analysed sample, authors state that they had the same risk profile for MI and the same sex ratio as the patients with a gold standard. In fact, they were more likely to be aged less than 40 years and hence less likely candidates for MI. Still, there is no information about 15 patients. Does the lack of data on gold standard on the 15 patients invalidate the results? We can test this by doing a sensitivity analysis. Assuming they were all protocol test negative but gold standard positive (worst-case scenario), we can recalculate the likelihood ratios (They turn out to be LR +11, LR −0.34)
What are the results?	
What likelihood ratios are associated with the range of possible test results?	LR for positive test result is 13.9, and LR for negative test result is 0.03. Presenting the results at three or more levels would have been more informative

(continued)

Guide	Comments
How can I apply the results to patient care?	
Will the reproducibility of the test result and its interpretation be satisfactory in my setting?	Standard test kit for CPK-MB is available. Authors give description and source of the assay they used. The description and source of the monitor for ST segment monitoring is also given. Both sources appear reliable. It may be desirable to have a quality control programme for the laboratory. Calibration and consistency checks should be run for both the tests on periodic basis
Are the results applicable to my patient?	Consecutive patients with chest pain were included in the study. They are unlikely to be systematically different from the population of patients with chest pain any clinician meets in emergency room. Therefore, the results are likely to be applicable in most settings. However, if authors presented the risk profile and other demographic variables of the study population, readers could determine the similarity or otherwise with their own patient population with more certainty
Will the results change my management?	Yes, depending on test results the patients will be admitted or discharged. The observation period for majority (82 %) of patients would reduce from 24 to 6 h
Will patients be better off as a result of the test?	To determine definitively whether patients are better off with the test protocol, one needs to randomise those coming to emergency with chest pain to receive or not receive the 6-h diagnostic protocol test. We could follow up the two groups of patients and compare the outcomes like cardiac failure, arrhythmia, time to remission of chest pain, deaths and patients' satisfaction. This would cover not only MI but also other causes of chest pain like acute pericarditis and dissection of aorta. This study focuses only on MI, but does not mention the duration of the chest pain and whether any other causes were diagnosed. Absence of this information limits the usefulness of the results
Are the likely benefits worth the potential harms and costs?	Yes, the benefits of 'ruling out' MI and consequent early discharge (hopefully after relieving the pain) are obvious. The costs of the test are likely to exceed the cost of unnecessary 24-h hospitalisation for most of the patients. However, the exact balance of risks and benefits would be determined only by an RCT

Comments on the scenario: Our patients had two risk factors for MI – age and hypertension. The pretest probability of his having MI may be around 10 %. If he is negative on the 6-h rule out test protocol, the posttest probability (with LR –ve = 0.03) is 0.33 %. This is clearly low enough to confidently discharge him. On the other hand if he is positive on the test protocol, his posttest probability is 60 %, which clearly warrants admission and further test to confirm MI and further management.

Critical Appraisal Questions for a Therapy Paper

Scenario: You are following a 55-year-old male with atrial fibrillation and history of transient ischaemic attack. He is on regular warfarin treatment. In one of the follow-up visit, his INR is 8. On checking, you find that he has not taken any extra dose of medication. You are worried that he may develop bleeding complication. You immediately ask him to stop warfarin. Your resident asks: Should we have a policy to give vitamin K to achieve early decrease of INR? You tell him, this is a good question. Why don't you find out the evidence for your question and discuss with me? (What is the clinical question?) He brings the following paper to you and you start evaluating the paper

Reference: Crowther MA, Julian J, McCarty D, et al. Treatment of warfarin-associated coagulopathy with oral vitamin K: a randomized controlled trial. Lancet. 2000;356:1551–53.

Validity assessment (Is the information likely to be valid?)	
Question	*Answer*
1. Was there a control group?	Yes
2. Was the control group created through concealed random allocation (randomisation)?	Yes, this is a randomised control study, but issue of concealment is unclear, because whether vit. K and placebo were provided in identical packs is not mentioned
3. Were the groups comparable (similar) at baseline?	Roughly, yes. However, placebo group is at some disadvantage because of older mean age and somewhat higher INR on day 0. This is unlikely to invalidate the conclusions
4. Was the initial balance maintained (through equal care to both groups and compliance)?	Yes, the primary outcome was observed 1 day after drug administration. Therefore, there was practically no chance of unequal care. Also, the drug and placebo (only one dose required) were administered under observation, and thus, compliance was ensured
5. Was the follow-up complete/ adequate?	Three patients (two from placebo and one from vit. K arm) did not turn up for follow-up, but this is unlikely to affect the conclusions. Even with worst-case scenario the difference in treatment success will be 11/46 (24 %) in placebo versus 25/46 (54 %) in vit. K; risk difference = −30 %
6. Correct outcome measurement (was outcome measured by blinded assessors?)	Probably yes. It is likely that laboratory measurement is not influenced by previous INR. Lab personnel were probably unaware of whether drug or placebo was to a given patient
7. Was the analysis based on intention-to-treat principle?	Strictly speaking, No. But it was not possible and does not invalidate the results
Results assessment (What is the information?)	
8. Did the new treatment make any difference in the study? (What is the magnitude of the treatment effect?)	Yes. In the reported analysis a risk difference of −36 %, NNT = 3. RR = 0.36; RRR = 64 %. Even with worst-case analysis, the RD = −30 %; NNT ≅ 4. RR = 0.44; RRR = 66 %
9. Is the observed difference unlikely by chance (*P* value)?	Yes, *P* = 0.001 indicates that the observed difference is most unlikely to be due to chance

(continued)

10. What is the study's margin of error (CI)?	Point estimate is very much on the left, and CI is entirely on the left as well. This indicates there is clear evidence that vit. K helps achieve acceptable INR earlier than the placebo
Applicability assessment (Can I apply the information to my patient care?)	
11. Is the study population relevant to my practice? (Can the results be applied to my patients?)	Yes
12. Is the intervention relevant (available, feasible and affordable) to my practice?	Yes
13. Is the comparison relevant to my practice?	Yes
14. Are all clinical relevant (important) outcomes considered?	Yes, both the favourable and adverse effects were considered. It appears that there are no significant adverse effects
15. Are the likely benefits worth the potential harm and costs?	Yes

Resolution of the scenario: After evaluating the evidence, you feel satisfied that the policy of giving vitamin K to patients with very high INR is safe and effective. Though you feel that there is probably only one randomised controlled trial, you would have been happier if the finding was confirmed by another group of workers. While you decide to look for more studies to support the conclusions of this study, you also decide to institute the policy of giving vitamin K to patients with very high INR and revisit the issue as and when you find more studies on the topic.

Critical Appraisal Questions for a Meta-Analysis Paper

Scenario: You are head of the medical services at your hospital. You are concerned that patients with stroke are not adequately cared for in the general medical wards. When the wards are full of acutely sick patients with myocardial infarction, pneumonia, hepatic coma, etc., then patients with stroke are relatively paid little attention. You approach the administration to establish a stroke unit in your hospital. As there is no neurology department in your hospital, you decided to look after all the stroke patients in view of your recent training fellowship in stroke. The administration asks you to provide evidence that stroke units can save lives and decrease the percentage of disabled patients. (What is the clinical question?) You search the medical literature and find the following paper, which you decide to critically appraise

Reference: Langhorne P, Williams BO, Gilchrist W, Howie K. Do stroke units save lives? Lancet. 1993;342:395–8.

Validity assessment (Is the information likely to be valid?)	
1. Did the review (meta-analysis) address a focused clinical question?	Yes, population, intervention, comparison and outcomes are mentioned, but a clear statement of the question would have been better
2. Was the search for relevant studies comprehensive and well documented?	Partly yes. The search terms are not mentioned. EMBASE is not searched
3. Were the included studies of high methodological quality?	Unclear. A section devoted to methodological quality is absent from the reports, but some points related to quality assessment are reported in the results section. Eight trials are reported to have a formal method of randomization, but how many had concealed randomization is not clear. Blinding is not a major issue because of impracticality of doing it and choice of a 'hard' outcome such as 'mortality'. Six withdrawals from stroke unit arm and 14 from control arm are unlikely to invalidate the conclusions. Assuming all of them to be alive is probably unwarranted, but as authors point out, this only strengthens the results because bias due to this assumption favours the 'general ward', in spite of which, in the end, the stroke unit arm fared better
4. Was there a good agreement between reviewers in selection and assessment of studies?	Unclear. No agreement statistics is provided
Results assessment (What is the information?)	
5. Were the combined results combinable (similar from study to study)?	Yes, the point estimate in Fig. 1 is reasonably close to each other. 955 CIs are overlapping. Tests of heterogenicity were nonsignificant – all favouring similarity of results from study to study except one study by 'Peacock' in Fig. 2
6. What are the overall results of the study (magnitude and precision of treatment effect)?	The meta-analysis showed an odds reduction of 28 % in mortality in the first 17 weeks and 21 % in the first year. The numbers corresponding to confidence limits of 95 % CIs are not provided, but visual inspection of the figure shows the limit near the null value line rather quits close If the true effect is so small in reality, then cost-effectiveness of stroke unit needs to be studied

(continued)

Applicability assessment (Can I apply the information to my patient care?)	
7. Is the study population relevant to my practice? (Can the results be applied to my patients?)	Yes. However, mean age of over 70 years indicated slightly older population than that seen in developing countries. It is unlikely, however, that the results would be remarkably different in the developing country population
8. Is the intervention relevant (available, feasible and affordable) to my practice?	The intervention has not been fully described. In all the studies, the intervention group comprised a specialist multidisciplinary team with an interest in stroke rehabilitation. Forming such mobile team is feasible. To develop a geographically defined stroke unit requires support from hospital administration
9. Is the comparison relevant to my practice?	Yes, very relevant
10. Are all clinical relevant (important) outcomes considered?	No. Functional outcomes are not analysed because of, according to the authors, the variety of outcome measures used
11. Are the likely benefits worth the potential harm and costs?	Can't say. Probably there is no potential harm, but cost-effectiveness is worthwhile to study

Resolution of the scenario: The paper appears methodologically sound. However, whether the stroke units are cost effective is not clear from this paper. Your administration demands that you produce papers demonstrating cost-effectiveness of stroke units. You decide to do more searches and appraisal of studies available on this topic.

Index

K. Prasad, *Fundamentals of Evidence-Based Medicine*,
DOI 10.1007/978-81-322-0831-0, © Springer India 2013

S

T

V

Printed in the United States
By Bookmasters